Ha
Hashimotos's Diet

An easy step-by-step Guide for
For fixing the Root Cause of
Hashimoto's Thyroiditis

Sabrina Wondraczek

Published in Germany by:

Stefan Corsten
Mürrigerstr. 9
41068 Mönchengladbach

This document is geared towards providing exact and reliable information in regards to the topic and issue covered. The publication is sold with the idea that the publisher is not required to render accounting, officially permitted, or otherwise, qualified services. If advice is necessary, legal or professional, a practiced individual in the profession should be ordered.

From a Declaration of Principles which was accepted and approved equally by a Committee of the American Bar Association and a Committee of Publishers and Associations.

The information provided herein is stated to be truthful and consistent, in that any liability, in terms of inattention or otherwise, by any usage or abuse of any policies, processes, or directions contained within is the solitary and utter responsibility of the recipient reader. Under no circumstances will any

Table of Contents

Book Description

If you're suffering from Hashimoto's disease, then it's fairly certain that you might have experienced a significant reduction in the overall quality of your life, from its symptoms to the horror of rapid weight gain along with the puffed up face look. You might even have found yourself wishing that you were more in control and who doesn't want to be in control, especially when it comes to your body and appearance? You now have the opportunity to gain back all the joy in your life by simply following these carefully selected techniques to not only master your hormones but also to lose weight. "Guide for Fixing the Root Cause of Hashimoto's Thyroiditis" is a comprehensive guide for your condition.

We are well aware of the suffering people that suffer this illness are bearing. If you have Hashimoto's disease, we are also aware of the struggle you are experiencing and most of all, the hard work you are putting in to get yourself out of this situation as early as possible. That is what we are here for—like a friend, to pat your back and give you advice you can hopefully use to achieve a better quality of life once more. The book you are about to read is especially on the topic of nutrition for Hashimoto's sufferers. The book offers a brief and easily understandable way of gleaning all the information required to fight this monster of Hashimoto's in the next days, weeks and months. To be clearer: when it comes to nutrition, it will only take 30 days of your life to feel the effects of what you're integrating right now! That means that 30 days could make a world of difference.

The 30 days that you take now to act against the disease, the 30 days that would make you suffer but not alone, and the 30 days that will take a great deal of your hard work and willpower will be worth the effort. But remember: You will feel the effects after 30 days, and earn the reward for all the hard work you'll put in. You do need to follow the instructions implicitly and we have included full information on your illness, so that you can understand the significance of your actions.

Here is a quick preview of the categories you should be expecting to be informed about, during the reading of this book, i.e., "Cracking the Hashimoto's Code - Hashimoto's Diet - From suffering to thriving in 30 days":

The book will guide you in terms of Hashimoto's diagnosis and the treatment that should follow. You can now gain control of your condition and life in general. Here's a little preview of what you should expect to learn from this book:

Hashimoto's Disease and Causes

Diagnose Yourself-Signs and Symptoms of Hashimoto's Thyroiditis
Conventional and Alternative Treatments for Hashimoto's

Effective Techniques to Shed Your Hashimoto Weight

Why diet plays a part in recovering
Diet Plan to Gain Back Your Energy
Dietary Causes of Hashimoto's.
Foods you should avoid.

Diet that contains essential nutrients to improve your condition.

Lifestyle Interventions you should take.
Best recipes to enjoy a Hashimoto's friendly diet.

Introduction

I want to thank you and congratulate you for purchasing the book, The New Hashimoto's Diet – An easy step-by-step Guide for fixing the Root Cause of Hashimoto's Thyroiditis.

This book has actionable steps and strategies on how to manage your thyroid condition so that you can feel healthy and vibrant again. You are probably concerned about being diagnosed, although the book puts everything in clear terms to give you a better understanding of your illness. We know that doctors sometimes talk in riddles and that's where this book goes one step further – helping you to get beyond the riddles to a real possibility of healing.

Are you always feeling tired even when you have not done anything to make you tired? Do you have muscle aches and pains? Are your muscles weak making it hard for you to engage in some strenuous activities? Do you have pale skin that is dry and have a puffy face? Have you recently gained weight even after consistently maintaining your calorie intake and daily activity levels? Do you experience drowsiness, eye pain and even depression? Do you have a large and lobulated thyroid gland? Not all of these symptoms will relate to Hashimoto's but are common to sufferers. This book will be able to help you to gain a better understanding of the problem and that's what it's been written for – for people like you who are looking for answers.

We all live in a polluted world now, where, hyperbolically and ironically speaking, more discoveries are made on diseases than on the species of animals existing on this planet. The more the world has progressed, the more it brought with it its advantages and disadvantages. Who knew that the invention of the refrigerator or the automobile could play a role in creating diseases? Yes, with all these inventions, human beings have not just gained advantages, but many of these advances have also been to blame for illnesses which are common in these times. For example, the pollution caused by automobiles has created illnesses such as asthma, migraines, high blood pressure, etc.

The food we eat on a daily basis is not what we, as a species, were naturally accustomed to consuming. Add pollutants, pesticides and all the additives and colorings contained in modern food and then consider today's hectic lifestyle. Human beings, because of their sedentary lifestyles are getting too little exercise. Top that with the lack of sleep common to many people, we've got a recipe for disaster.

Hashimoto's disease is the most common form of the thyroid gland inflammation. This disease is not a monster unless you make it one, but by taking no precautionary measures and by not even considering your own doctor's advice, you may be making the monster worse than it has to be. This need is, in fact, to gird up your loins and get this business sorted out before it is too late. If you have any of the symptoms that you will find in our symptom checking chapter, then visiting the doctor is common sense. He will be able to diagnose your condition and then you will know if this eating plan is going to be useful to you in helping you to come to terms with your illness and overcome all of the ill effects that it causes in your life.

We have laid out a dietary plan in this book – in fact we have referred to two so you have the choice – so that you can use diet to improve your condition easily and without too much inconvenience. That's right! Patients can control their condition with diet. The link between diet and Hashimoto's is well established and accepted in the scientific world.

Are you aware that around 20 million Americans have a thyroid disorder? The worst part is that only 7 million have been diagnosed. This means that many people are walking around experiencing the inconvenience of symptoms and living miserable lives when they could do something about the situation. While Hashimoto's thyroiditis is treatable, it is the lack of adequate information about thyroid diseases and disorders that has meant that many people still live in pain, when they really don't have to.

Despite its common nature, Hashimoto's disease isn't actually very well known among the masses. There are those who continue to remain misdiagnosed or without any diagnosis all of their life despite having traces of this disease. This book will provide you with all the necessary information valuable for you to not only understand the disease, but also to diagnose it. Obviously, the last say in all of this will be your doctor's, but oftentimes you have to suspect the disease beforehand in order to get yourself checked or tested for that matter. When you do, there comes a certain peace of mind because it's acknowledged that you have a problem and it is then that you can treat it and change your lifestyle to accommodate the inconvenience and indeed to overcome it.

This book series is aimed to guide you on your way to improve your Hashimoto's condition, and to get rid of its symptoms by following the advice given in the chapters that lie ahead.

There is only so much that your doctor can tell you. Of course, doctors are trained professionals with all the right experience and knowledge. Those with specialization in the field of Thyroid disease are experts of Hashimoto's, but these experts often lack time to teach you every little detail about the disease. You may even forget to ask the right questions. Moreover, doctors tend to stick to the scientific aspects and treatment for every known disease, and if you're looking for alternative approaches then you might require a different resource. This book series is a bit of both for you. Not only does it cover every important detail, but also alternative diet plans and treatments as well, giving you more choices.

The natural remedies offered would offer you the kind of choice that you truly deserve and can be used apart from the prescribed medication. When you take control, diseases such as this don't have to take over your life. After all, Hashimoto's is treatable; this makes it something that is within your power and control. We think that your body weight and facial appearance should not be decided upon by the apathy of doctors, whose only recourse is to dose you up with Levothyroxine. This helps to stabilize your levels, but there's so much more that you can do.

It is quite common for the medication to cause facial swelling, and reduced your energy. However, with the diet plan and energy gaining techniques described here, you will be able to feel at your best once again. The extra weight you put on can now be controlled and reduced quite effectively so it isn't the end of the world. The information contained in the book does in no way imply that you do not to listen to your doctor, but actually enhances your overall insight relating to this particular disease. It offers you an alternative way of dealing with your weight and overall appearance, along with gaining a sound control over your energy levels.

Firstly, we are going to talk about the symptoms and signs of Hashimoto's and later, we will discuss the imbalance of hormones that the patient of Hashimoto's experiences. Lastly, we will give you most of the treatment you should undergo while suffering through Hashimoto's. In between, we will be looking at diet and nutrition and I have even given you some ideas for recipes that you can try. You may wonder why diet is so important to patients. That is explained as well and you have the choice of which diet suits your purposes better.

This book will help you understand more about your thyroid and Hashimoto's thyroiditis, which is a condition that affects the thyroid gland. You will learn about the common causes of this condition as well as the role that your diet and eventually your gut play in this condition. You will also learn how to deal with the problem from its root causes, which is diet and get the freedom from the discomfort of this disorder. Thanks to this book, you no longer need to suffer from Hashimoto's thyroiditis and will better understand your body and its needs. Scientists and doctors agree that with a healthy gut you can have a healthy thyroid and vice versa, so dealing with the root cause would seem to be a very common sense way to move forward.

What is the Thyroid?

The thyroid is a hormonal gland essential for the regulation of major processes in the body that include metabolism control, growth and maturation. The thyroid helps regulate these processes by releasing hormones into the bloodstream at a steady rate; more hormones are released when the body is in need of greater energy, like during pregnancy or in the winter season. This is something that normally gets done as a matter of course during your life and in people who do not suffer Hashimoto's is an automatic reaction of the body's mechanisms.

The gland is made up of 2 lobes, each about the size of half a plum; they are joined together by a ridge of tissue known as isthmus. The two lobes are found on both sides of the windpipe, with the gland as a whole located just below the voice box or Adam's apple. Chances are that you will be unaware of this gland from feeling your neck, unless it has formed a goiter. In fact, its presence is quite discreet, and although you may think that something this small cannot play such an important role in the body, you need to understand that indeed it does.

A thyroid gland weighs 20 to 60 grams on

average and is encircled by two fibrous capsules; the outer capsule is connected to a bunch of muscles and highly important nerves. A loose connective tissue sits between the capsules so that the gland can physically move when a person swallows. The tissue itself is made up of a number of individual lobes that are joined together by a thin sheath of tissues.

The thyroid is responsible for producing three hormones, namely:

Triiodothyronine or T3
Tetra iodothyronine, also called thyroxine, or T4
Calcitonin

T3 contains three atoms of iodine while T4 contains 4 atoms of iodine; T4 is converted into T3, which has a wide control over activities going on inside the body's cells. These hormones regulate the speed of cells, i.e. the speed at which they work. If the hormones are secreted too fast, the cells start working at a higher rate than would be normal and a condition known as hyperthyroidism develops. This would mean an increase in the heart rate in some cases so is relatively important. On the other hand, if the glands work too slowly, then the body suffers from hypothyroidism. Hyper means overactive and hypo means underactive. This is made obvious from the readings that a doctor gets from a simple blood test.

Since these hormones are so important, they are usually stored abundantly in the body; some are stored as droplets while others are tied to carrier proteins. When the body needs these hormones, they are released from the proteins. In addition to T3 and T4, the third hormone known as Calcitonin is responsible for proper bone metabolism in the body.

As the hormones are responsible for raising the body's metabolism rate, they:

Raise the body's temperature,
Make the heart beat stronger, raising the pulse,
Break down food in the liver at a quicker rate and thus energy is supplied at a faster rate as well.

Promote growth,
Promote brain maturation,

Activate the nervous system, which leads to higher level of attention and concentration.

However, the thyroid shouldn't work too fast

either as that would be unhealthy. Here's a table that shows the various effects of an overactive and an underactive thyroid. You will see from this that the activity of the thyroid is quite vital to good health and can affect many bodily processes that are diverse in nature. For such a small part of the body, the thyroid has a huge role to play in controlling all of these activities and actions of the body.

Overactive thyroid	Underactive thyroid
Trembling	General loss of energy
Weight loss	Tiredness
Hot flashes	Being overweight
Sweating	Slowed metabolism
Hair loss	Constipation
Diarrhea	Difficulty concentrating
Nervousness	Slow pulse
Insomnia	Dry skin
Restlessness	Loss of sexual

	desire
Fatigue	Deep hoarse voice
Racing heart	Waxy skin

As it was mentioned earlier, in the first chapter, Hashimoto's thyroiditis causes the thyroid gland to work at an underactive rate, therefore the person usually suffers from the symptoms of hypothyroidism. Not everyone will suffer from all of the symptoms shown, but these are common. You need to note that these can also be symptoms of other things, so that it is necessary to get confirmation from your doctor if you believe that you have Hashimoto's disease symptoms.

How is Thyroid Activity Measured?

Your doctor will be the point man in this case and he/she will be able to make an accurate assessment of your situation by looking at your symptoms or through a physical exam.

Otherwise, you may use the symptoms list given in a chapter below to self-diagnose the thyroid disorder known as Hashimoto's thyroid. Be a little careful with self-diagnosis as the range of symptoms is diverse and could be related to other ailments. If you suspect that you have it, the next step is to actually have this diagnosed properly through a doctor.

What is Hashimoto's Thyroiditis?

Hashimoto's is officially known as Hashimoto's thyroiditis in the world of science. It is among the most common forms of inflammation of the thyroid gland. The inflammation of your thyroid gland is termed thyroiditis. Hashimoto's thyroiditis is the most common disorder related to the thyroid in the United States. It is also called autoimmune thyroiditis, which is what most patients tend to call it. Another common scientific name for the disease is chronic lymphocytic thyroiditis. This is the most popular name among doctors.

Before we can even start looking at the treatment of Hashimoto's thyroiditis, it is important to have a comprehensive understanding of what it is. Hashimoto's thyroiditis is a disease where your immune system attacks a very small gland known as the thyroid gland, which is located just below the Adams apple (at the base of your neck), which is explained fully in the last chapter. This gland is important to your body since it coordinates many of the activities in the body including metabolism, growth and development. Inflammation of the thyroid gland caused by the onset of Hashimoto's disease (also called chronic lymphocytic thyroiditis) causes the thyroid gland to become underactive. Owing to the female sex genes being more prone to thyroid disease as well increased physical, emotional and mental stressors placed on women, the condition is more common in women. However, this does not mean that men cannot suffer from Hashimoto's disease. It is just higher in prevalence in women.

Surprisingly enough, the disease actually affects about fourteen million citizens in the United States, which is an important enough statistic to make you realize the chances of you or a loved one having it or getting it at some time in your life. As you can imagine from the name of the disease, it has a Japanese origin. A Japanese surgeon who was the very first individual to have discovered it in the year 1912 basically inspired the name of this disease. The disorder is basically autoimmune in nature. This means that your body's immune cells, which are meant to protect or defend the body against foreign cells, begin to attack the healthy tissues within your body instead of offering protection.

This attack is not due to any deficiency or incorrect behavior by the healthy tissue, but rather a mistake being made by the immune cells. The process of attacking these healthy tissues is what causes the inflammation of your thyroid gland.

Interestingly, your gender actually decides your chances of getting this autoimmune disease to a certain extent. Women tend to be more likely to be affected by this disease. According to the latest statistics, women are seven times more likely to be diagnosed with this particular autoimmune disease as compared to men. This figure is backed up by Healthline.com and many other health websites and for the sake of convenience, I have added links in full at the end of the book.

When the malfunctioning occurs, the immune cells of your thyroid gland experience the attack, and this causes impairment of your thyroid gland. It impairs the gland's ability to produce one of the most significant hormones of your body; your thyroid hormones! Reduced production of these hormones causes a condition known as hypothyroidism. Basically, when the autoimmune disease causes severe enough attacks to your thyroid gland to such a point that it loses all of its ability to produce thyroid hormones, then your whole body loses its ability to function properly. This is when most people with Hashimoto's develop hypothyroidism. Should you be concerned at that description? In a way, yes and in other ways no. People live long and healthy lives with Hashimoto's disease once they have it under control, though you should be aware of changes that happen and report these to your doctor.

Don't think there's no trouble coming your way just because you don't have hypothyroidism, as it is definitely not the sole complication that can be associated with Hashimoto's disease. There are certain cases, though not very common, where the Hashimoto's thyroiditis causes the gland to become inflamed to such an extent that it over enlarges in size and the development of a goiter is achieved as a consequence. However, you will know when this happens and are likely to seek medical help. One thing that you should rest assured of is that the goiter is relatively slow growing and does not impede your breathing. It should however be checked out as soon as it appears as this is something that is usually benign but should not be ignored.

One thing should be clear to you that once your body develops an autoimmune disease then your immune system is bound to malfunction one way or the other. Some of the most common autoimmune disorders include:

- Addison's disease

- Type 1 diabetes
- Rheumatoid arthritis

If you already have an autoimmune disorder, then it is probably time for you to check for the development of Hashimoto's thyroiditis. Your natural risk factors for this particular disease may be higher compared to a normal individual without any autoimmune disorder. Doctors and experts suggest that you should consider getting yourself checked for Hashimoto's more often in order to remain safe. Your doctor will determine how often you should be getting yourself tested.

Why would you need checking several times?

Since Hashimoto's disease is an evolving disease, there may be times that you feel that there have been changes in your symptoms and may need more or less medication. Thus, a blood test will be ordered by your doctor which tells him all about the TSH levels, as well as giving him readings of T3 and T4. TSH is nothing more sinister than Thyroid Stimulating Hormone and T3 and T4 are explained in a later chapter.

There are many ways for you to detect the symptoms of Hashimoto's disease, which will be discussed further in the book. Now that we have a better understanding of what Hashimoto's thyroiditis is, I know that you are asking what causes this condition.

Causes of Hashimoto's Thyroiditis

You are now aware of the fact that Hashimoto's thyroiditis is in fact inflammation of your thyroid gland. Do not take the condition lightly, as the thyroiditis has the potential of destroying the entire thyroid gland if it is left untreated. However, if treated, it is simple to keep it under control and even to adjust your lifestyle to lower the incidence or inconvenience of thyroiditis.

The scientific name for the immune cells is lymphocytes. Hence the scientific name of Hashimoto's: chronic lymphatic thyroiditis. These lymphocytes not only destroy the tissue in the gland after entrance, but also the blood vessels and the cells within the thyroid gland. Moreover, the entire process of destruction of the thyroid gland is quite slow. This is the reason behind undetected Hashimoto's thyroiditis in many people. What does seem to bring these out of hiding is the fact that the symptoms are tiresome and patients are likely to seek medical advice for the side effects during which blood tests may reveal the presence of the condition.

The symptoms are also quite vague, and take

time in becoming noticeable, which is why you have to keep a look out for them, especially in case of a pre-condition of an autoimmune kind. The disease is not dependent on the complete elimination of the thyroid hormone. Even the reduction in the hormone will stop the body from functioning normally, which ultimately leads to hypothyroidism – not to be mistaken with Hyperthyroidism which is an overactive thyroid.

The body's immune system is designed to defend your body against any viruses and bacteria of a harmful nature, but what makes them turn against the healthy tissues is not entirely certain until now. However, there are certain risk factors associated with this disease that scientists believe are the causes of this disease. These factors include the following and need to be taken into consideration when assessing if you may be suffering from it:

Poor Diet

This is actually one of the main causes of this condition. We will have a look at this closely in a later chapter. In addition to a poor diet, other things could be linked to Hashimoto's. Gut health is important and thus what you eat is equally as important. You also need to keep yourself hydrated and drink a lot of water but that's good for other things as well. Your diet is vital to your condition and cutting out convenience foods should be your first port of call. You know from there being so much information available what these foods are that need to be cut out, but we deal with the actual suggestion of different diets to control the disease later. If you have only read as far as this, look through your cupboards, because much of what you have in the larder will probably be convenience foods with additives and many different chemicals that are not that good for your overall health.

Family Background

People with Hashimoto's thyroiditis are more commonly those with family members who have various kinds of autoimmune diseases and other forms of thyroid diseases. This clearly suggests that a genetic component plays a certain role in this particular disease. It mostly affects the HLA-DR5 gene. If you know, for example, that your parents or siblings have had to deal with this condition, you may find that you have it too or could suffer from it at some time during your life. It is a wise precaution to keep in touch with your family on health matters because all of the details that you glean can be useful to you in the future, regardless of whether they are concerned with this or other illnesses.

Some Infectious Diseases

Some diseases and some drugs can trigger the disease in already genetically predisposed individuals. Examples of the diseases are Turner, vitiligo and Down's. Fungal infections of the nails and the mouth can also cause the disease. If you have suffered from any of these, do consult your doctor, who may be able to distinguish whether what you suffered from is related to Hashimoto's.

Hypoparathyroidism

This is a condition whereby your body secretes abnormally low levels of parathyroid hormone.

Hormonal Causes

As mentioned earlier, Hashimoto's disease is more likely to affect women as compared to men, which suggests the role of your sex hormone in this as well. Moreover, it is commonly observed that women have thyroid related issues during the first year after having given birth to their first child. Though these issues generally fade away, there are still as many as 20 percent of such women who end up having developed Hashimoto's after a certain number of years.

Some of the hormonal problems that can cause this condition include adrenal insufficiency and type 1 diabetes whereby the hormone insulin does not function as it should. Estrogen fluctuations in the presence of genetic susceptibility can also trigger the disease.

Since hormonal activity is likely to be associated to Hashimoto's this may also occur if you have had a hysterectomy because the levels of hormone are likely to change. Other events that may trigger Hashimoto's are menopausal changes, when Hashimoto's is likely to kick in because of those changes.

Aging can have an effect in both men and women – women for obvious causes of changes affecting hormones and men as a consequence of aging. As previously stated, more women suffer from it than men to, though women over the age of 65 account for a rise in the percentage of women having the illness to 20 percent.

Excessive Iodine

Research has suggested that there are certain drugs that contain iodine or taking excessive quantities of nutrients can cause the triggering of thyroid disease in people who are susceptible. Excessive quantities of iodine is another reason people may develop Hashimoto's. Thus it's important to be certain about supplements that you may take as part of your daily routine. The danger is that people take too many of these and depend upon them every day of their lives when in fact, there is no natural need for them, since the body can produce many of the minerals that people take already.

Radiation Exposure

The cases of thyroid diseases have been increased in those who have more exposure to radiation, especially in countries like Japan. Moreover the radiation treatments for Hodgkin's disease (a form of blood cancer) have also been known to cause thyroid diseases. Research has backed this up and patients who have had radiotherapy in the neck area have an increased chance of developing

Hashimoto's. (2) There is a link at the end of the book to support this assertion, written for the US National Library of Medicine.

Pregnancy

Pregnancy can also affect the thyroid. Some women have thyroid problems after having a baby, but these usually go away. But there is a significant ratio of women who developed Hashimoto's after going through pregnancy. This percentage is about 20% of these women who developed Hashimoto's disease in later years. Again, the link to hormones is clearly visible from the causes drawn up in this chapter.

Other Diseases

There are certain kinds of patients who are more commonly found to have been misdiagnosed with some other disease due to similar symptoms. Such diseases include:

- Chronic fatigue syndrome
- Depression
- Anxiety disorder
- PMS (Pre-menstrual syndrome)

- Fibromyalgia
- Cyclothymia

The reason behind such a misdiagnosis is that while in the initial stages of hypothyroidism, the symptoms tend to be comparatively non-specific. If you have been treated for any of them, there is a certain amount of guesswork based on the doctor's experience of your health record and assumptions made can be incorrect. If you doubt your diagnosis, do not hesitate to ask your doctor for a blood test.

The problem is that the aches and pains do give the impression that you are suffering from something that is related to arthritis or chronic fatigue, but you may find that you do not respond to the treatment that you are given and get frustrated by the lack of apparent improvement.

As far as depression goes, if you feel that your problem is deeper than simple depression, running blood tests is a wise move because it may save you from taking medication that is not geared toward your illness. There may be slight improvements in humor because of the raise in levels of serotonin, although if the problem comes from Hashimoto's, that improvement may only be temporary.

As you can see from the above, the causes for Hashimoto's are varied and thus this accounts for why the problem is often hard to pinpoint. However, if you are frustrated with treatments being ineffective and have to visit the doctor's office on a regular basis, it may be worthwhile mentioning if you think that you may have thyroid problems, especially if you know these to be in your family history.

Signs and Symptoms of Hashimoto's Thyroid Disease

Hashimoto's reveals its symptoms very gradually. The signs and symptoms can be mixed up with other diseases, considering the fact that they are quite vague. It is very easy to misdiagnose a person with Hashimoto's, unless you have confirmed the diagnosis with the aid of laboratory tests. At a very basic level, there are certain symptoms that are a characteristic of a patient with this autoimmune disease. Whenever a doctor suspects that someone is suffering from Hashimoto's, these are the signs that he will be looking for. Did you recently experience one or more of the following? If so, you may be suffering from Hashimoto's and it may be worthwhile asking your doctor what he/she thinks.

Fatigue and Sluggishness

Fatigue and sluggishness are very common signs of Hashimoto's disease. This can be explained very easily because in this disease, the blood level of free t4 is very low and due to this, your metabolic rate is also very low. Hence, the body is deprived of enough energy even to undergo even the daily activities.

Some people may feel tired and lethargic all the time. If you take a look at the Hashimoto's patient's lifestyle, you will often realize that they have not indulged themselves in anything that could deplete their energy reservoirs. However, most patients still feel short of energy - so much that it becomes a serious problem for them to complete their daily tasks properly. They may also be lethargic and wonder why their life seems to be devoid of energy when they have done nothing energetic to explain it.

Puffy Face

Having a puffy face is also one of the characteristic features of this lethal autoimmune disease. This is one of the symptoms that a lot of people find really hard to tackle. There are two primary reasons for this symptom. First, there is a condition called myxedema in which there is fluid retention in the body. The reason behind this retention is that the tissue fluid is not adequately cleared from the body. When the tissue fluid does not get cleared out properly, then it starts to accumulate and eventually causes swelling that is visible to the naked eye. In the case of myxedema, the swelling is mainly under the eyes and on the extremities as well.

This leads to puffiness of the face, which becomes very obvious after a little while. The second reason for this is that in all the autoimmune diseases, the function of the kidney is impaired. Due to this impairment, metabolites and tissue fluids are not excreted in appreciable amounts and hence fluid retention becomes a very obvious feature one can expect when suffering from one of these autoimmune diseases. In certain cases, the edema is so exaggerated that even diuretics can't really fix it completely. Those are some rare cases otherwise in general when the hypothyroid condition gets cured, and then edema also gets lessened to the maximum possible extent. If your hypothyroidism is caught early enough and take appropriate treatment, this may not affect you, so do not think that everyone suffering from Hashimoto's disease will suffer this symptom.

Unexplained rapid weight gain

It is very commonly seen that people who are suffering from Hashimoto's disease undergo a massive increase in their weight, which is completely unexplained considering their appetite is no different to normal. This is also one of the very innate features of this disease. The reason behind this is a lack of thyroid hormones in your blood. As you might already know, thyroid hormones are responsible for regulating the metabolism of the body. If there is a lack of these hormones in your body, then your basal metabolic rate will be slowed down to a great extent.

When your metabolic rate gets really low, your body doesn't utilize all the energy that it is being provided with. Owing to this fact, there is excessive fat deposited in your body, and that leads to the weight gain that the Hashimoto's patient experiences. The alarming factor in this situation is that the weight gain is extremely rapid, which wouldn't be possible under normal circumstances. Hence, you need to pay attention if you have gained a lot of unexplained fat lately.

The weight gain occurs infrequently and it rarely exceeds ten to twenty pounds. Most of the weight gained is in form of liquid. You may notice bloating particularly in the gut area and this is explained later in the book as this is very relevant to the disease and the diets that are suggested for sufferers of this disease. Do not ignore it because fat deposited in these areas can impede the function of essential bodily processes.

Stiff joints

This disease makes your joints stiff and painful. The small joints on your hands and feet also swell. Knee joints may also swell. This shouldn't be taken as an indication that you have Hashimoto's disease on its own, since it may signal other illnesses such as arthritis or arthritis associated illnesses.

Muscle aches

Hashimoto's disease also causes tenderness and stiffness of the muscles causing muscle aches. The most affected are the muscles on the hips and shoulders. Quite frequently this will improve with treatment and it is likely that your doctor will look for other causes if this persists.

Prolonged and excessive menstrual periods

For women, Hashimoto's thyroiditis prolongs your menstrual bleeding leading to what is known as menorrhagia. However, since many women have their Hashimoto's diagnosed after menopause, this will not affect them in this way and refers to younger patients.

Muscle weakness

People who suffer from this disease might also complain of muscle aches throughout their body. The reason behind this is that people who are suffering from this condition have an accumulation of lactic acid in their body, which causes tenderness and pain in the muscles. Lactic acid needs to be broken down and gets removed by the body, otherwise it causes pain in your muscles and stiffness in your joints. Diet can help you to prevent this pain. In particular, bananas are good for helping to dissolve the excess lactic acid, as well as increasing your intake of bicarbonate since this adds alkalinity to offset the acidic effect of the lactic acid. You have to remember with Hashimoto's that your body is not functioning to its optimal levels and your diet should compensate for any deficiency.

Pale skin

This condition makes your skin pale and dry and gives you a puffy face. It might also make your hair and nails dry. Not everyone will suffer from this, although it's always a good idea to make sure that you have a great care routine for your skin anyway which will help dryness as and when it occurs.

Hoarse Voice and Depression

People who have this disease sometimes experience hoarseness. There is a difference between a normal heavy voice and an abnormally hoarse voice. If you see a case with the latter, then you need to pay attention to the patient because this is also one of the signs of Hashimoto's. The reason for this and partly for the depression is that a patient may feel that he/she cannot swallow correctly and this seeming constriction of the throat causes the voice to alter pitch. Not being able to swallow can also cause anxiety that can in turn lead to depression.

Sensitivity

Due to the extremely low rate of metabolism, the people suffering from this disease feel cold at temperatures that are completely normal for other people. This is owing to the fact that the metabolic activity going on in your body is responsible for the homeostasis- maintaining a constant internal environment. People suffering from this disease might always feel cold even at ordinary temperatures. This is due to the fact that in any normal case, your body maintains a constant temperature by making alterations in your basal metabolic rate. There is also the tendency to be unable to cope with overheating as well when your electrolytes become affected. The problem in this case is lack of potassium and diet can fix this and get your electrolytes back in action. As a measure for safety purposes, it would be a good idea for patients to keep electrolyte treatment that is used for kids in their homes as this is very effective and brings the levels back to normal together with a good balanced diet.

Drowsiness

In addition to feeling drowsy, you may also have a hard time in concentrating on whatever you are doing at a particular time. However, this can also be put down to tiredness and you must make sure that you have sufficient sleep for your body's needs.

Firm, large and lobulated thyroid gland

This can be due to lymphocytic infiltration. If you have an enlarged thyroid gland, then it is worthwhile visiting your doctor since your thyroid may have a goiter.

Eye pain

The pain can be so bad that you experience some difficulty looking at lights. The reason for this is the closeness of the pituitary gland to the eyes and since this works hand in hand with the thyroid, this is common.

Constipation

Constipation is not, as such, a sign that is going to stay there constantly, but it has been observed that Hashimoto's patients suffer from it on and off. In case you are suffering from this condition, you must at least consider Hashimoto's as one of the possibilities. This is owing to the fact that when your basal metabolic rate is really low, then that also decreases the peristaltic movements of your gastrointestinal tract. When the movements of the GIT get decreased, then the bowel movement also does not remain very adequate. This leads to constipation and the person might feel bloated or experience abdominal cramping. Be very careful not to misdiagnose constipation. A lot of people do and simply treat this with over the counter constipation meds, but this could be a mistake because it can lead to a lazy bowel and a constipation habit.

The symptoms are many but some of them could be due to other factors or other minor diseases. Ensure you go for a periodic check-up of your thyroid if:

- You have ever had thyroid surgery
- You have had any kind of radiation therapy to your upper chest, head or neck
- You have had treatment with anti-thyroid medication or radioactive iodine
- If your family has had a history of thyroid disorders
- If Hashimoto's thyroiditis is not treated early, it can lead to several problems like:
- Severe heart problems and even heart failure in extreme cases
- Thyroid cancer
- Decrease in libido
- Seizures, coma and eventually death
- Severe dyspnea, which is shortness of breath
- For pregnant women, it could lead to a miscarriage

This is a general regime of symptoms that might

appear in patients but will not all appear. Similarly, it is not necessary that every patient who is suffering from this disease must have all these symptoms. It has also been seen that some people have a lot of these symptoms but they have a normally working thyroid, so the important thing that you need to remember is that you should always consult your doctor if you are encountering any of these symptoms, even if thyroid is not suspected. You can only be sure about your condition if it has been proved by a laboratory diagnosis. When you go to the doctor and tell him about your symptoms, he is going to advise some tests that you have to undergo in order to get a proper diagnosis. Thus, for the sake of a simple blood test, it is certainly worthwhile checking it out as this can save a lot of worry and the test really is not invasive at all. Another test which may be ordered if you are found to have Hashimoto's is an ultra sound exam which is very easy to undergo. This is where a technician holds the ultra sound reader against your skin, to read any anomalies, so this is not invasive either.

Imbalance of Hormones in Hashimoto's Patients

There are three major hormonal imbalances that people suffer from during Hashimoto's disease. In this area of the book, not only we will teach you about these hormones, but also offer some hints about what you can do to rebalance them. However, all the treatments will be discussed in detail in the next chapter.

The thyroid is one of the glands that make up the endocrine system in the body. Screwing up the thyroid will ultimately screw up the whole of your endocrine system, and all of the hormones it produces. The thyroid produces and stores hormones and releases them into the bloodstream as and when they are needed, and from there, they are carried to the parts where they are required. These hormones are released, and then travel through the body and direct the activity of the body's cells, which are waiting for their orders.

The two master hormones that the thyroid produces are:

triiodothyronine (T3)

thyroxine (T_4)

The thyroid makes two types of thyroid hormones: triiodothyronine (T_3) and thyroxine (T_4). T_3 is the active hormone working in your body, whereas T_4 is the precursor. T_4 levels need to be sufficient to produce enough T_3. There are a number of things that these thyroid hormones have the control over, which are as follows:

- Metabolism
- Brain development
- Breathing
- Heart and nervous system functions
- Body temperature
- Muscle strength
- Skin dryness
- Menstrual cycles
- Body weight
- Cholesterol levels

Other hormones control these thyroid hormones—these other hormones are thyroid-stimulating hormones (TSH), which are made by the pituitary gland in the brain and regulates thyroid hormone production.

If one ceases to perform its function, the other ultimately fails too. When thyroid hormone levels in the blood are low, the pituitary releases more TSH and likewise, when thyroid hormone levels are high, the pituitary decreases TSH production. Thus each of these measures are vital to perfect health and will be the measures that are taken during a blood test.

You can see from this list that the thyroid function is necessary to a lot of the important bodily functions and thus if the levels change and do not supply the needed T3, problems arise.

Explaining the Relationship Between T4 and T3

During diagnosis and treatment for Hashimoto's Disease, you will be given blood tests but it's a good thing to know what these mean and what can be read into them. Your doctor will see straight away if you have hypothyroidism and is likely to opt for standard medication for the disease. However, knowing what T4 and T3 stand for can help your understanding of the condition and to appreciate how serious the role of the thyroid is in all kinds of bodily activities.

When you are suffering from Hashimoto's what it means is that there is an imbalance in the T4 and T3 hormones that are circulating in the system. So what are these and what do they do? When doctors explain things to a patient sometimes they forget that the patient has no real understanding of all these numbers and letters and that's why we feel it is vital for you to understand in plain English. The standard medication for Hashimoto's is T4 or levothyroxine. Although patients who suffer from Hashimoto's may feel that this will help, it may not address the balance between the T3 and T4 levels since it doesn't actually mean that the conversion rate between T4 and T3 will be balanced. There are all kinds of things that affect this and you need to see the fuller picture because to a certain degree, you control that balance and this control can be by the diet that you eat.

Let's try and split this into the different reasons why conversion is not happening and look at some areas where you can help it to happen.

Mineral deficiencies

When you don't have a good balance of minerals in your body T4 doesn't convert to T3 and you can address this quite easily by finding out if you have a deficiency in zinc that is the most likely cause of problems. Getting tested is the first step. Take things slowly and methodically because the way that the body works is very complex. Introduce too much of something or assume that you don't have enough zinc and you may just be causing more problems than you should. Ask your doctor to test your zinc levels but before taking on other advice, get the overall picture from other potential causes of imbalance.

Gastrointestinal problems

These may affect the absorption of the correct minerals and may be the cause of the imbalance between T3 and T4 but often doctors don't look at this side of the equation. This is where you need to examine your diet and help yourself as much as possible to balance the levels.

Insulin Imbalance

People suffering from Hashimoto's may also suffer from insulin and blood sugar imbalances, which can lead to diabetes. Low thyroid function can cause dysglycemia and metabolic syndrome through a variety of mechanisms. Let's see what a thyroid dysfunction would cause in your body:

- it decreases the rate of glucose absorption in the gut
- it slows the response of insulin to elevate blood sugar
- it slows the rate of glucose uptake by cells
- it slows the clearance of insulin from the blood

When you are hypothyroid, your cells aren't very sensitive to insulin, so even though you have normal levels of glucose in your blood, you may experience symptoms of hypoglycemia. These symptoms are: fatigue, headache, hunger, irritability, etc.

We have gathered all the symptoms that would signal you if there is any kind of hormonal imbalance in your body:

• Bloating
• Bone loss
• Irregular periods
• Irritability
• Loss of muscle mass
• Loss of scalp hair
• Low libido
• Memory lapses
• Mood swings
• Nervousness
• Night sweats
• Poor concentration
• Sleep disturbances
• Tender or fibrocystic breasts
• Urinary incontinence
• Vaginal dryness
• Weight gain
• Decreased fertility
• Depression
• Excess facial and body hair

- Hot flashes
- Heavy or painful periods

Just as soon as you observe your body showing signs as such symptoms given above, go to your doctor and have yourself tested in order to save yourself from serious consequences. In fact, even if you do not have Hashimoto's or a serious Insulin imbalance, the peace of mind that can be achieved from the blood tests will be worthwhile.

Testing for Hashimoto's Disease

Hormone Test

This test is conducted in order to check the level of certain hormones in your body. Those hormones determine the activity of thyroid gland. The tests are for TSH (thyroid stimulating hormone) T4, T3, and fT3. All of these give your doctor an idea of what is going on with your thyroid.

TSH Test

TSH is the thyroid-stimulating hormone. When a person's thyroid gland is impaired, then it doesn't produce the normal amounts of thyroxine. When there is not enough thyroxine in the blood, then the body demands it, and sends messages to the brain, telling it to produce more thyroid stimulating hormone which is adequate enough to stimulate the thyroid gland to producing more thyroxine. Now, when the thyroid gland is malfunctioning, then it will still not produce any thyroxine despite being stimulated by a large amount of thyroid stimulating hormone. Now, due to the lack of the thyroid hormone, the body will keep on sending signals to the brain, and it will keep on producing a large amount of thyroid stimulating hormone. As this will keep on happening, we will see an increase in the level of thyroid stimulating hormone in the blood. This is one of the determining factors for Hashimoto's. It must be taken very seriously if your serum TSH levels are elevated. This is a major problem if that's the case. A healthy level of TSH is 0.3 and is 3.5 mIU/L with Hashimoto's patients. It's not uncommon to see levels in the range of 4.5 mIU/L or above than that.

T4 Test

In order to check the level of thyroxine in the blood, laboratories basically check the level of thyroxine (T4) in the blood. This is considered a very important diagnostic character for showing Hashimoto's disease. The level of T4 in the blood will be very abnormally low. This is due to the malfunctioning of the thyroid gland. Even though the level of TSH is very high in the blood and the brain is continuously giving signals to the thyroid gland to produce thyroxine, the gland is unable to catch that signal. Healthy levels of T4 are 4.6-12 ug/dl while with Hashimoto's patients, it's not uncommon to see levels in the range of 14 ug/dl or above.

Free T3

This test measures the free T3 hormone levels. This test is rarely recommended by doctors, and it is usually only used when the patient shows some symptoms of hyperthyroid and his fT4 levels are normal. Note we said hyper which means overactive. Nonetheless, if you are suffering through Hashimoto's, you might want to know the amount of active thyroid hormones. Therefore, this test can be really useful in this regard for finding out what amount of active thyroid hormones are present in your body for the thyroid receptor sites. FreeT3 aka Ft3 is high in hyperthyroid conditions, but it is low in hypothyroid conditions. Also, it may be high in thyroid toxicosis. 230-619 pg/d is the normal range of fT3. In any condition i.e., Hashimoto's, it moves from this limit to 700 pg/d or above.

Free T4

This test, Free T4, is used to measure the amount of free or active T4 in the blood. For Hashimoto's patients, it is highly recommended because if you leave it a bit late for this test, this might cause the T4 to lose control and worsen the situation. FreeT4 is high with hyperthyroidism, but it is low with hypothyroidism. There is a drug called Heparin that can cause elevated free T4; just like that, some acute illness can also cause elevated free T4. The normal range of Free T4 is 0.7-1.9 ng/dl. Hashimoto's is caused when it exceeds this limit. You may be prescribed Heparin for other problems so make sure that your doctor is aware of why you are taking it and what other medications you take, as well as the dosages.

Reverse T3

You need to test your Reverse T3 level, which is usually produced when there is an extreme amount of stress or anxiety or sudden shock. For example, a severe car accident or a chronic bout of stress could be a cause of this.

When the body produces high amounts of the stress hormone cortisol, this is elevated; and also as a stress response, it is elevated. But when is it low? In a condition when one has severe tissue damage such as a severe burn or diseases like cirrhosis, etc. Normal rT3 level is 0.11 - 0.32 ng/ml in adults. A fluctuation from this range, mainly "above" this range, will cause Hashimoto's.

The relationship between T3 and T4 and what it means to bodily function

For T3 to exist, you need T4. T4 actually gets activated as and when the body needs it. T3 contains 3 iodine atoms and T4 contains 4. These work in conjunction with most of the systems within the body and are therefore vital to normal function. Thyroxine is T4 and if you have Hashimoto's you do not produce enough of it which means that you need to up that level by taking the drug Levothyroxine. T3 levels are controlled to a certain extent by the action of the thyroid gland to send messages to the pituitary gland that more TSH is needed which is produced by converting T4 into T3. Thus the relationship between the two and the balance of these hormones is vital to the function of the body. If T3 is in short supply, the metabolism is affected and if the T4 gets in short supply, there is nothing to top up the needed T3. Many of the diets work on the premise that they produce the much needed iodine into the diet that triggers the action needed to make the body more efficient. T3 and T4 circulate within the blood and diet counts here because proteins carry it. Laboratories measure T4 free as well because this equates the T4 that is ready for conversion. The free T4 test usually goes hand in hand with the blood work done for establishing if the thyroid is out of synch and helps the doctor to determine where the problem lies.

Iron

Iron is very important for every human being, but especially for people going through Hashimoto's. Women usually complain about their iron level. So here are a number of tests that you need to undergo in order to check the level of iron:

Serum Iron is necessary for making hemoglobin in your body. Its function is to carry oxygen in red blood cells. A decreased level of iron must be correlated with RBC, HTC, and HGB to exclude anemia.

TIBC, which is an abbreviation of Total iron binding capacity, is an elevated in iron deficiency because, as the test name suggests, it increases the cells' potential to bind iron. It is high before anemia develops in your body, which ultimately can be a way to find iron deficiency sooner.

Transferrin is an iron absorption regulator. It is increased with iron anemia. Its test will preferably give a hint of iron's level in your body.

Ferritin is a very helpful marker for total body iron levels. It gives a detail of how much iron the body has stored. It also known as an "acute phase reactant," and thus it is a good marker of inflammation. Normal range: ferritin - 45 (22-322).

The normal hemoglobin range is 13.5 to 17.5 grams (g) of hemoglobin per deciliter (dL) of blood for men, and generally it is 12.0 to 15.5 g/dL for women. Iron, serum - 193 (40-155) is the range you'll get after the test. You need to keep the level of iron balanced in your body in order to prevent Hashimoto's. The entire dietary plan that you need is given in the second book of this series.

Ask your doctor for a test for your iron levels as this may be useful in finding out what your diet lacks as this could be important. As we will state and restate throughout this book, Hashimoto's can be controlled by diet and paying attention to dietary needs is vital. Make sure that you talk to your doctor about your results and speak to him/her about improving those levels.

Antibody Test

Due to the fact that Hashimoto's is an autoimmune disease, there will be an abnormally high production of antibodies. This is again a very characteristic feature of Hashimoto's disease. The test is going to reveal a very high amount of antibodies against thyroid peroxidase. Thyroid peroxidase is an enzyme that is normally present in the thyroid gland, and it plays a very important role in maintaining the normal activity of the thyroid gland. It is very important for the production of thyroxine, and any anomaly in the production of this enzyme will also lead to a great deal of loss of the production of thyroxine. That's something that needs to be addressed.

There are three types of antibodies that are tested, which are given below:

Thyroid Peroxidase Antibody (TPO Ab)
Thyroglobulin Antibodies (TgAb)
Thyroid-Stimulating Hormone Receptor Antibody (TRAb)

Thyroid Peroxidase Antibody (also, abbreviated as TPO Ab):

This antibody is the one that is mostly high in autoimmune thyroid conditions such as Hashimoto's. It is also called a microsomal antibody. Less than 35 IU/mL causes Hashimoto's in its patients.

Thyroglobulin Antibodies (abbreviated as TgAb):

Thyroglobulin Antibodies aren't very often seen as high as TPO Ab. Preferably, they are ordered only when thyroid lab results do not give a definite result because these antibodies are also suspected as interfering with thyroid hormone production.

Less than 20 IU/mL can cause Hashimoto's.

Thyroid-Stimulating Hormone Receptor Antibody (abbreviated as TRAb):

This antibody--thyroid-Stimulating Hormone Receptor Antibody—is only ordered when a patient is hyperthyroid. When it gives a positive result, the patient is suspected of having Grave's disease. 1.75 IU/L or less can cause trouble.

Selenium Test

We have already discussed in the previous chapter the working of selenium in your body, and from that discussion, you might have concluded that selenium deficiency may influence both the immune response as well as the peroxidation of thyroid cell components, thus making it a very important factor of controlling Hashimoto's in your body. Thus, in case you are feeling the signs of Hashimoto's in your body, what you need to do next is, after your doctor's suggestion, to have a selenium test on your body. You have to keep checking until you feel a normal, healthy environment around you. The current DV (Daily value) for selenium is 70μg (micrograms), which is quite fit for every individual. Also, you need to keep this in mind that every dietary product that you use daily has a different amount of selenium in it. Therefore, it is best to consider the amount of selenium in these products before their usage.

We cannot emphasize enough that reading labels really does help your diet and you should be aware of dietary goodness at all times when you have Hashimoto's disease because with the right nutrition, you really can control this disease.

Vitamin D Test

You must consider a vitamin D test after you have seen the signs of Hashimoto's in your body. This test is, however, important for you to be taken during and after Hashimoto's, so that you do not get to see any trouble later. Patients with Hashimoto's thyroiditis presented lower levels of vitamin D inversely correlated to antibody levels and directly correlated to thyroid volume. Thus we can say that there is a relation between vitamin D deficiency and the development of Hashimoto's thyroiditis. Normal levels of vitamin D vary from 50-80 ng/mL.; and anything below 32 contributes to hormone pathway disruption. Most people are deficient in this critical vitamin, so get your Vitamin D Levels checked with the help of your doctor or a home testing kit. Vitamin D is also very necessary for your bones and you need to ask your doctor what you should avoid eating and drinking when taking it. Certain foods and drinks will affect its efficiency in the body.

Ultrasound

An ultrasound uses a device called a transducer that bounces safe and painless sound waves from organs, and then creates an image of their structure on a screen. A specially trained technician performs the procedure in a health care provider's office, and the doctor interprets the images. These images taken from the ultrasound can show the size and texture of the thyroid, as well as a pattern of typical autoimmune inflammation, which would directly help the health care provider verify Hashimoto's disease. It may also be used to see if there is a goiter forming on the thyroid gland.

CT Scan

A CT scan uses a combination of x-rays and computer technology to create images of the diseased part of the body. For a CT scan, the patient may be given a solution to drink and an injection of a special dye called contrast medium. Then the CT scans requires the patient to lie on a table that slides into a tunnel-shaped device where the X rays are passed. The patient does not need anesthesia. In Hashimoto's disease, a CT scan is used to examine and analyze the placement and extent of a large goiter, and then to show what affect the goiter has on nearby structures. This will only be done in cases where the ultra sound has found a problem or where the patient is experiencing a serious problem that the doctor feels should be investigated further.

As I had earlier indicated, there is a very close relationship between Hashimoto thyroiditis and your gut health. Let us look at this close link so that we can be able to treat Hashimoto from its root cause, which is diet.

Conventional and Alternative Treatments and Tests for Hashimoto's

Conventionally, the most ideal choice for the treatment of Hashimoto's is levothyroxine. This is the drug that is being used most commonly all over the world.

Levothyroxine

Levothyroxine is the drug that is most commonly used for the treatment of Hashimoto's disease. Its route of administration is oral, which makes it easy for the patient to consume. The dose is given once daily because it has a comparatively longer half-life, and hence it stays in the blood for a longer duration. It takes a little while for the medication to show an effect, and thus for the patient to get back to the steady state. Levothyroxine treatment is a lifelong intervention because it doesn't treat the root cause but rather the symptom - low thyroid hormones.

Now there are also alternate ways for curing Hashimoto's. These work more on the root of the problem, rather than its symptoms and I will be going into more detail later on in this book. For now this is just an overview:

No Caffeine and Sugar

It can be beneficial to prohibit yourself from having a lot of caffeine or sugar in your diet. This also includes all forms of refined sugars such as flour. Your main focus should be to eat non-starchy vegetables and meat, as we will discuss in the second book of this series. If you really cannot give up coffee, then you need to drink it in a decaffeinated state. Sugar substitutes such as saccharin are ill advised and it is far better to get sweetness from the fruits that you eat, rather than taking sweeteners.

Protein Content

It is very important to increase the protein content in your diet. Proteins are responsible for transmitting thyroid hormones at cellular level in your body. Things that you can have for protein are fish, meat, and eggs, for example. If you lack protein, the thyroid hormones may not be able to be transmitted efficiently and this can make the condition worse.

Fatty Food

It is a common misconception that fat is bad for health. You need to understand that not all kinds of fat are bad for your health. Cholesterol, for example, is really important for a lot of hormonal processes, and thus the metabolism in your body. Lack of cholesterol can lead to hormonal inadequacy that can also apply to your thyroid hormones. You will also need to add foods such as olive oil and avocados, which are more mono unsaturated fat, as well as coconut products for MCTs and cholesterol, and fatty fish for Omega 3s. If you are unaccustomed to using this kind of product, now is the time to change. Saturated fats are the harmful ones and you need to learn the difference.

Micronutrients

This may not be a primary reason for Hashimoto's, but if micronutrients are very inadequate in your diet, it can further aggravate the already present symptoms in your body and make your condition worse. Hence, it is especially important to have vitamin D, zinc, selenium, copper, iodine, vitamin A, and vitamin B. Looking for foods which are rich in these is therefore essential, rather than simply carrying on with an unsatisfactory diet and taking dietary supplements.

No Gluten

The molecular composition of thyroid tissues is similar to that of gluten, which is why people suffering from this disease should completely stop having gluten in their diet! This is a very important step, which we will discuss in detail in the second book of this series. However, if the food you are eating can be mistaken for thyroid tissues, it's quite likely that you will suffer from leaky gut as a consequence of having too much gluten.

Avoid Goitrogenics

Certain foods that cause goiters should be completely taken out of the diet. These foods include turnips, spinach, cabbage, sprouts, millet, Brussels sprouts, watercress, soybeans, rutabaga, radishes, peanuts and peaches. You don't have to leave them out altogether but it's better to avoid them to the greatest extent.

Get More Glutathione

Glutathione is a powerful antioxidant that

strengthens the immune system, and it is extremely important for your body to fight against this disease. It helps in giving your body more energy to regulate the immune system. Some foods help your body in producing glutathione. They include garlic, grapefruit, raw eggs, whey protein, and avocado. Cauliflower is also a very safe option, and asparagus can also be considered for this purpose.

Restore your GUT FLORA

Thyroid functioning is also dependent on healthy bacteria that are present in your GI tract (GIT). What you should do is feed yourself with friendly bacteria. Those probiotics help to increase the quantity of these bacteria. Kimchi and Kefir are good sources, and you might consider a probiotic supplement as well. This is vital when you have this illness because without helping your gut, you can become prone to leaky gut. This is when your gut is allowing impermeability. You can use glutamine to help to line the stomach but it's a far wiser precaution to address your diet.

The Common Misconception about Iodine

It is believed that an inadequate quantity of

iodine leads to Hashimoto's, but this is not the case. It has been proven that if you take iodine supplements when you already have this disease, then it is going to make the condition worse. You just may want to add iodine to your normal diet, and do not take any special supplements for that. There are primary and secondary sources for that. The primary source of iodine is seafood. Secondary sources on the other hand include eggs, asparagus, mushrooms, spinach, garlic, sesame seeds, and summer squash. That is why these foods were suggested in a previous chapter and in a natural state taken through food, the body can manage the amounts introduced much better than if you decide to take supplements that worsen the situation.

Vitamin D3 is Key

Exposing your skin to natural sunlight creates Vitamin D3. Therefore, it is advisable to get some responsible sun exposure every day. If you're deficient in Vitamin D3 as indicated by blood testing, it can also be a good idea to supplement your diet with 5.000 – 8.000 iU of Vitamin D3 daily until you hit optimal levels. The range of illnesses that are affected by vitamin D3 is diverse and this should be taken seriously. Natural sunlight is essential to life.

Omega 3 for a Healthy Immune System

Omega-3s, which are found in fish, grass fed animal products, flaxseeds, and walnuts, are the building blocks for hormones that control immune function and cell growth. These are very important for proper thyroid functioning, and this is going to enhance the ability to respond to the thyroid hormones. Omega 3 is good for other things as well so you won't be wasting your time making sure that you have sufficient in your diet. For example, Omega3 spreads are healthier than butter. The importance of fish, especially oily fish, cannot be over-estimated since this really does help your immune system immensely.

Low Level of Selenium

Selenium is also an essential element for the conversion of T4 to T3, which are selenium-dependent. Selenium works as a deiodinase enzyme, the enzyme that removes iodine atoms from T4 during conversion. As I've explained before, low T3 can cause hypothyroid symptoms, as it is the active form of thyroid hormone. According to a study, it was found that selenium supplementation in selenium deficient patients modulated T4 levels, supposedly by improving peripheral conversion to T3. When the body has a severe deficiency of selenium, the conversion of T4 to T3 may be impaired, thus leading to hypothyroid symptoms. To keep a check on the level of selenium in your body, it would be advisable to take a blood test. Make a note of the supplemental blood tests that would be useful and have these at the same time to save yourself the inconvenience and expense of running separate tests.

Homeopathic Treatment for Hashimoto's

I have added this because it may help you. There are several homeopathic medicines that are used to treat Hashimoto's disease patients and these help to restore a little of the balance within the body to make the patient feel that their body is more in control. The particular medicines that are used are *Calcarea Carbonica, Sepia Officinalis, Lycopodium Clavatum and Graphites* but the most important ones are Calcarea Carbonica and Lycopodium Clavatum because the first deals with the imbalance within the body and helps the patient with the side effects of Hashimoto's while the second is wonderful for digestive tract problems. Do not self-medicate. If you do choose to go this route, then you need to find a homeopathy practice that is well established, so that they rather than you decide upon the quantity you are given. You can expect fairly rapid results, but you need to look after your diet to keep your Hashimoto's in check that is why we have given you a choice of two diets that will really help you.

Lifestyle Alterations to Help Your Hashimoto's

Starting from the beginning of time, everything that humans possessed, consumed, and did was much simpler than it is these days. The environment we live in now can be hazardous to our health. Most of us suffer from a lack of sleep, constant stress, and low activity levels. A better lifestyle is just a few simple steps away, and it will help you in fighting your condition. Here are the interventions for you to take. There is a chapter to help you with sleep that may be useful to those who find sleep difficult. Since this is essential to good health, you really need to take it seriously as part of your daily regime.

(a) 1: Have some sun exposure

Do you know how important Vitamin D3 is? Without it, your immune system can become unbalanced, and its deficiency can lead to an expression of an autoimmune attack on the tissues in your body. Therefore, to avoid deficiency, we advise you to get some responsible sun exposure daily. If this means just walking down to the road to the corner shop, do it. If you are not that active, try to go outside into the yard so that you have sufficient daylight. It isn't enough to be sitting in a sunny room. You need to ensure that you get your exposure on a regular basis, since you already have an immune disease.

(b) 2: Work out but don't over train!

Sometime Hashimoto's gets women thinking that their bodies are getting completely deformed by being overweight. What you'll need to do first is to relax and think wisely. If you want to exercise, then you should consider short sessions of weight training. On the other hand, chronic steady state cardio, for example jogging, may raise your cortisol levels. Getting your regeneration between sessions is important! Don't take on a strict regime of exercise all at once. Build up to it and try to be supervised so that you know your safe limits.

(c) 3: Let go of external stressors

Stress is good for us and we need stress, as long as it is intermittent and not chronic in nature.

Chronic stress wreaks havoc on your system, as it increases cortisol and promotes inflammation, as well as adrenal fatigue. Take breaks in your daily life, and de-stress yourself with the help of meditation. We have included a section in the same section as we have included covering sleep as this may be useful to Hashimoto disease sufferers.

(d) 4: Sleep is necessary!

Why do we sleep? Why is it so important to sleep? The fact is if one does not sleep, it will cause the level of cortisol to get heightened and in return, your body will be disturbed mentally and physically, leading to a condition where you will have mood swings and you will make bad food choices. Also, a lack of sleep will disturb the blood sugar regulation in your body. Do read the chapter about changing lifestyle habits as this gives more detail on how to get sufficient sleep.

(e) 5: Ground yourself!

It might seem strange at first sight, but grounding is actually a concept that is well backed up by science. Grounding means putting yourself in contact with the Earth. You can sit or walk barefoot in nature or use a special grounding mat while sleeping. Grounding has been proven to reduce cortisol and inflation markers. This is also known as Earthing and it has been found to be very beneficial to people with immune diseases and scientists are looking into the other benefits as they do seem to be far reaching. Walking down the garden path in bare feet can actually help you to recharge your batteries and if you disbelieve this theory, then it may be worthwhile reading a report on it that is written by Doctor Stephen Sinatra of the Heart MD Institute, a link for which has been provided at the end of this book.

Correcting Your Lifestyle to Include Meditation and Relaxation

I have included a section for this since is does play an important part in staving off an immune disease or the effects of it. We have already said that sleep is vital and that relaxation and lack of stress can also help. However, many people don't find it easy to sleep or to relax and meditate. This section is to help with this element of your Hashimoto's because it will benefit you long term to learn to relax and to learn how to get a good night's sleep. Quite often, people who do get Hashimoto's disease and who are suffering from hypothyroidism feel tired all of the time, but they don't achieve quality sleep. Instead, they veg out and are not active.

You do need to keep active as we have explained in the previous chapter, but you also need your sleep more than you can ever imagine. During the course of sleep, your body is permitted to heal and if you deprive your body of that sleep, you will feel sluggish and your body's natural defenses are unable to kick in and help you through your illness. Thus, learning to get to sleep is vital. There are several determining factors that may affect your sleep:

Is your bedroom geared to sleeping - or are there distractions such as a computer?

Do you watch late night TV that is fast and violent?

Do you ever read in bed?

Do you allow your mind and body to slow down ready for sleep?

Do you snack at night?

Do you drink too much coffee and tea at night?

The ideal way to prepare for sleep is to make sure that you are ready for it. Your bedroom should be a comfortable temperature. If it's too hot and your bedclothes are uncomfortable, you won't sleep easily. If you are too cold, you are equally taking away the feeling of wanting to go to sleep in favor of wrapping yourself up to keep yourself warm. You need a fresh atmosphere in your bedroom so air it daily.

Get out of the habit of drinking caffeine drinks at night and try instead to limit your intake of food and drink before bedtime. How can you sleep if you have indigestion or if you have just eaten and this has not had a chance to digest properly?

You need to take going to bed seriously and make sure that when you go to bed, you are not going to be distracted and indeed that you can stay in bed for the required hours to help your body to go through all the processes that sleep entails.

You can combine meditation and relaxation by lying in bed and closing your eyes. Think of nothing except your breathing and the body part that you are concentrating on. Think first of your feet – flex them and feel them flex and then relax them. If you are in the habit of thinking things through last thing at night, try to get out of the habit because your subconscious mind is capable of chewing things over and giving you answers in the morning once you allow it to. Think then of the next part of the body, working from your feet up to the top of your head, tensing the area and then relaxing it, until your whole body is relaxed. Chances are that if you do this at bedtime, you won't get that far and will simply fall asleep.

The relaxation that you afford your body when you have Hashimoto's is important as it is with any autoimmune disease. You allow the body to heal from within when you allow yourself eight hours of sleep a night and this is vital to good health. This section is only small but the importance of rest cannot be overstressed. If you find yourself going back to thoughts during the relaxation process, start again at your feet because you need to get out of a very bad habit – thinking when you are supposed to be sleeping. A lot of the time, when you have Hashimoto's disease you will feel tired and sluggish, but you give your body more energy when you sleep correctly, eat the right foods and exercise sufficiently.

Meditation on its own is a little different, in that you sit with your spine straight and learn to concentrate on your breathing. You breathe through the nose, hold the breath for a short moment and then breathe out but that's not the all-important thing. Many people get lazy in their breathing habits and are not aware that they are being lazy. Breathing through the mouth is one bad habit, though swallowing too much air can also make the digestive system even more difficult than it normally is and can cause bloat. When you meditate, you need to rock the upper abdomen as you breathe in and out. This is the correct way to breathe and will take you a little time to achieve. However, meditation means that you think of nothing except the process of breathing and if you need to concentrate on something concrete, try to think of the breath as an energy entering your body, lingering a moment and then leaving. As you do this, you should think of nothing else, so having your eyes closed and being in a calm environment is very important.

Although you may not think that these actions can help you with your Hashimoto's they can. They help you to focus. They help you to gain energy and they also help you to have the right frame of mind to be careful in your lifestyle so that you don't make the illness worse than it should be. Remember the thyroid affects everything and if you can relax and concentrate on your meditation, you give your body a chance to properly digest food and your mind time to energize. Energy is probably what you are lacking, so you can see that there is indeed a link between Hashimoto's and meditation.

If you think that it will help you, by all means join a yoga club because you may find that you get more support and will stick to your practice, which will in turn help you considerably. The best thing about a class is that you are taught the right way to do things and will find it very beneficial.

Diet and Hashimoto's

As indicated in a previous chapter, diet plays a very important role in Hashimoto's disease. We will thus look at the various things in your diet that could be aggravating your thyroid gland. We will start from looking at gluten and its role in Hashimoto's. The link between Hashimoto's disease and diet is an established one and there is no question that changing your diet can improve your condition and make it easier to live with. It can actually make your Hashimoto's something that you no longer have to worry about because by mending your diet, you take control of your illness and that's very important to Hashimoto patients.

Gluten and Hashimoto's

It has been established that there is a very close relationship between gluten and Hashimoto's disease, such that if you are found to have Hashimoto's, you are tested for gluten intolerance. So, what is gluten? Gluten is a composite protein of gliadin and glutenin. Gliadin's molecular structure resembles that of the thyroid gland. So, when you take food rich in gluten, the gliadin is likely to breach the gut's protective barrier and then enter the bloodstream.

This is referred to as leaky gut. When the gliadin enters the bloodstream, the immune system releases antibodies to destroy this foreign body. Since gliadin is very similar to the thyroid in terms of molecular structure, the same antibodies that destroy the gliadin also start attacking the thyroid. Therefore, if you already have Hashimoto's or any other autoimmune thyroid disease, you need to stay away from gluten. As such, you ought to embrace a gluten-free diet because this kind of reaction and destruction of the thyroid gland can even last up to six months. Adopting a gluten free diet "occasionally" won't be enough; you need to ensure that your diet is 100% gluten free to prevent any autoimmune destruction of the thyroid.

Blood Sugar Imbalances and Hashimoto's

Your blood sugar levels can also trigger Hashimoto's and even make it worse. How is this so? When you take a diet high in carbohydrates, your pancreas will secrete insulin, which enhances the absorption of the glucose into the muscles. Over time and as you eat a diet high in carbohydrates, your pancreas has to secrete more insulin to deal with this. This means that with time, you will need more insulin for the glucose to be absorbed into the muscles. Research has indicated that continued insulin surges that are very common in insulin resistance can also lead to destruction of the thyroid gland if you are suffering from an autoimmune disease like Hashimoto's. As the thyroid gland is damaged, the production of thyroid hormone reduces. Thus, you find yourself locked into a vicious circle.

As much as high blood sugar is bad for you if you have Hashimoto's, so is low blood sugar. When you have low blood sugar, the adrenal glands produce a hormone known as cortisol, which informs the liver to produce more glucose in order to bring back the sugar levels to an acceptable level. Additionally, cortisol is the stress hormone that is responsible for the "fight or flight" response. This response usually leads to an increase in heart rate, which then increases the rate of blood flow to your muscles so that you can fight or flee from the danger. The problem with this is that continued cortisol increase, due to the low blood sugar levels, suppresses the pituitary function since the pituitary gland makes the thyroid-stimulating hormone that stimulates the thyroid gland to manufacture thyroxine. This means that if the pituitary gland is not functioning as it should, your thyroid also will not, which can make Hashimoto's worse.

Gut Bacteria and Hashimoto's

One of the many important functions of the good gut bacteria is to assist in the conversion of T4 into its active form T3. Usually, 20% of T4 is converted to T3 in the gastrointestinal tract into triidothyroacetic acid and T3 sulphate. The conversion of these two into the active T3 normally requires an enzyme referred to as intestinal sulfatase. This enzyme comes from healthy gut bacteria. Therefore, if you don't have these healthy gut bacteria, you are likely to have problems with your thyroid - in this case Hashimoto's.

Vitamin D deficiency and Hashimoto's

Deficiency of vitamin D has been associated with many autoimmune diseases including autoimmune thyroid disease. Vitamin D is very important as it usually regulates the secretion of insulin and blood sugar sensitivity. Research even shows that a deficiency in vitamin D can lead to insulin resistance and, as we saw earlier, blood sugar levels greatly affect thyroid function.

You may then think that by simply increasing the intake of Vitamin D, you will be okay. Well, it is not that simple as that as certain mechanisms can affect the production and reduce absorption of vitamin D in the body. We will have a look at some of these mechanisms:

- First, not eating adequate fat or not digesting fat, as you should, makes it hard for your body to absorb vitamin D since it is a fat-soluble vitamin.
- Since vitamin D is usually absorbed in the small intestines, when you have a leaky gut, this will reduce absorption of nutrients including the absorption of vitamin D.
- Any kind of inflammation reduces the utilization of vitamin D
- A number of drugs like antacids, blood thinners and anticoagulants reduce the absorption of vitamin D

Thus you can see that there are many elements that need to be brought into the equation to get the full picture. For example, did you know that taking vitamins with hot drinks might actually diminish their value? A lot of people take no notice of things such as this and expect their vitamins to do the job they are supposed to do, but caffeinated drinks can actually diminish the value of the vitamins taken. This you are strongly advised to avoid these.

You can also see that there are several drugs that have an interaction against the absorption of vitamin D and since many patients will be on these drugs, they need to discuss with the doctor how to get around the problem of having sufficient vitamin D. As people get older, they are more likely to be taking drugs for other medical conditions and this makes Hashimoto's patients in this age range less likely to have sufficient vitamin D in their diet that is actually getting to the body parts that need it.

As you have seen above, you cannot have a healthy thyroid without a healthy gut and you cannot have a healthy gut without a healthy thyroid. This means that to deal with Hashimoto's there is a need to address the gut and thyroid simultaneously.

This will be the topic of our discussion in a future chapter. First, we need to look at FODMAPS which may be an expression you have never heard of before, but which is very relevant to Hashimoto's Disease patients because of the link between the action of the thyroid and digestion. You do need to have a fuller understanding of this aspect because it may affect the way that your Hashimoto's disease responds to the food that you eat. As you are probably aware, fermentation takes place in the gut and you are told by adverts on the TV that you need to create a healthy balance whereby you have sufficient bad and good bacteria. This is where FODMAPS may actually be making your life more difficult, so they do need to be discussed in case they have a bearing on persuading you that it is time to change bad habits to help your gut to digest foods correctly.

What are FODMAPS?

It's quite complex but FODMAPS stands for Fermentable Oligosaccharides, Disaccharides, Monosaccharides and Polyols. Some of the foods within your diet are foods that contain carbohydrates. We all know that excessive carbohydrates are not a good thing to add to your diet, but if the sugar from the food that you eat is not digested, it can cause excess fermentation in the gut. So what's wrong with that? You may think that this would only cause you to have a bit of extra wind, but really it's more complex than that. A lot of people who have IBS and other gut problems cannot eat foods that fall into this category of foods because they produce too much pain and the potential to cause diarrhea.

FODMAPS are in foods that you might not suspect as being unhealthy, so in order to understand a little better, I have included a list of things that you need to avoid if you also want to keep your gut working in an effective manner. With Hashimoto's, your gut will need all the help that it can get to stay in good health, so this should be taken seriously. FODMAPS also have an effect on constipation and you may be surprised to learn that many of the things that you thought were healthy within your diet may actually be detrimental in the case of people with Hashimoto's disease, which is why we encourage people with this disease to use low FODMAP foods as an alternative to high FODMAP foods. A quick substitution and all your digestive problems could disappear very quickly indeed and that's valuable news for Hashimoto sufferers.

Everywhere you look on the Internet when you associate the word Hashimoto's with Constipation confirms that there is a very strong link between the two. The disease encourages constipation. Constipation is not only bad for you but it makes you feel so rotten as well and the excess fermentation that is taking place in your body is certainly not doing your body any good. It's a very risky business messing around with your digestion and people often associate this kind of fermentation to be an acid stomach. Not only that, the amount of over the counter medications that are sold to the public show that people are treating their condition themselves because they don't know any other way of coping with it. The fact is that self-treatment isn't working. In fact, in the case of Hashimoto's it could be making matters worse.

There is a link between common use of these types of medication with stomach tumors, less effective absorption and continued problems. Thus it can be seen that even if these give short term relief, they are unlikely to help long term and may be setting you up for even more trouble than you bargained for. The point is that you must treat the cause rather than the symptom and the cause is firmly in the types of food that you eat. If your diet consists of foods that fall into the High FODMAP range and you switch down to low FODMAP foods, you can improve your gut health enormously without resorting to unwanted medication. All it takes is a better understanding of what's happening to your gut. Although some of the foods in the high FODMAP range may seem healthy enough, in the case of illness, these are to be avoided because they are not helping the body and can easily be replaced with Low FODMAP foods that help the system to perform optimally.

Foods are also split into different areas so that you can instantly recognize that group of foods such as Lactose foods, etc.

(f) HIGH FODMAP FOODS

Dairy/Lactose

Food that need replacement:

- Yogurt
- Powered milk
- Milk
- Margarine
- Dairy desserts
- Soft cheese like ricotta
- Cottage cheese

Polyoils

- Cauliflor
- Pumpkin
- Snow peas
- Nectarine
- Lychee
- Cherry
- Prunes
- Plums
- Pears
- Apple and apricots
- Most attrificial sweeteners

Fructose rich

- Spring onions
- Radicchio
- Lettuce
- Leaks
- Garlic
- Asparagus
- Artichokes
- Chicory
- Beetroot
- Barley
- Rye and wheat (when in antity)

Legunes/Saccharide

- Soy milk
- Soy flour
- Baked beans
- Chickpeas
- Lentils
- Kidney beans
- Bortolotti beans

Fructans

- Figs
- Mangoes
- Pears
- Watermelons
- Corn syrup
- Sokids
- Agave
- Honey
- High fructose corn syrup
- Rum
- Pistachio
- Cashew nuits

Thus, you will see that there are conflicting stories to the ones that you are accustomed to hearing about the nutritional value of foods. FODMAPS that fall into the table below are low FODMAPS that help your gut to digest more easily and thus improve the function of T3 and T4 conversion. Thus your metabolism becomes better and you can correct a lot of the acidity that you are experiencing.

(g) LOW FODMAP FOODS

Dairy/Lactos

- Lactose free milk producs
- Ice creams
- Sorbets
- Hard cheeses
- Such as cantal and cheddar
- Parmesan
- mozzarella

Polyoils

- Blueberry
- Grapefruit
- Banana
- Honeydew melon
- Passion fruit
- Raspberries
- Strawberries
- Kiwi
- Grapes

Fructose rich

- Lemons

- Lines and all fruit containes in the previous column
- Maple syrup
- Table sugar

Legumes/Saccharid

- Firm Tofu

Fructans

- Gluten free bread
- Cakes
- Biscuits etc. (red Labels)
- Beansprouts
- Bell peppers
- Chives
- Eggplant
- Lettuce
- Sprouts
- Green beans
- Spinach
- Potato
- Bok choy
- Bean sprouts

- Carrots
- Tomatoes
- Iols
- Containing infusions of onion or garlic
- Gluten free cereals
- Rice cakes
- Corn pasta
- Potato chips

You do not have to deprive yourself, but make simple adjustments to diet to avoid the high FODMAP FOODS as this really will help your health. The diets that we have chosen at the end of the book are those which do this and which introduce healthy foods for Hashimoto's sufferers. You will see that there are some surprises in store for you when changing over from High FODMAP foods to low ones and you may find that you actually get to prefer them and don't feel deprived when you find the foods that are good replacements. Read labels on breads, cereals etc. because this is where a lot of mistakes are made.

Remember that table sugar in small quantities is better than using sweeteners. That may surprise you but what happens with sweeteners is that the sugar high is short-lived and that leads your body to wanting more sweeteners that makes a vicious circle. Since sweeteners are BAD FODMAP foods, this may be where you are going wrong and this small adjustment may make the world of difference.

No one is expected to cut out all of the high FODMAP foods, but this chapter is more to help you to be aware of the load that these have on the digestive system so that you can lower the load and feel the benefits of changing your diet to one which has less high FODMAP foods at each meal. You will feel the benefit of this if you are suffering from digestive problems as a result of your Hashimoto's. In fact, using FODMAP foods has helped a very high percentage of people who also suffer illnesses such as IBS.

Introducing a New Diet

In this book, you will see that we have taken two approaches to using diet as a means to improve your condition. There are basic differences in the approaches given, one being more radical than the other and a requiring a lot more discipline and the other system being something that you think of in the long term because it's more a way of life than simply a diet. The two choices were obvious ones from the point of view that they are both relevant to sufferers of Hashimoto's and it's worthwhile reading through the different diets and seeing which one you believe you would be able to follow and stick to bearing in mind that you want to gain maximum benefit from your diet. Remember that this isn't just about diet. It's about diet, exercise and sufficient rest, as well as drinking plenty of fluids.

You will know to what extent your Hashimoto's is affecting you but if you want long term results that are likely to last, the Paleo is perhaps the best option because this allows you to have a more efficient digestive system while incorporating all of the protein necessary to retain good gut health long term. You will also more effectively lose weight and get your thyroid back into balance. The shorter term solution, i.e. the GAPS diet is a good solution for those needing proof that this kind of diet can help them in their quest to be healthier even though they have been diagnosed with this illness. Before we start on each of the diets, we will give you an overview of the approach so that you will be much more able to adhere to the diet. Preparation is everything when you are changing the habits of a lifetime and this preparation will explain what the diet does, why you are on it and the long term benefits of it on your health. Your approach to diet is as important as your daily intake because if you leave too much temptation in your way, this will hinder your progress and may just tempt you to cheat.

Introducing the GAPS Diet

This diet is interesting because the mistakes that people make when they replace foods with what they believe to be better alternatives are sometimes what is getting in the way of progress. What better demonstration can I give you of the control you begin to take of your life than to look at the case of one successful user of the GAPS diet? The reason that people are looking for alternatives is that the variety of symptoms that they are getting from Hashimoto's are so diverse that they put people in a situation where they feel they lack control over their own wellbeing. Some of the symptoms that this lady suffered from were very worrying indeed and traditional medicine had failed her. The symptoms are varied because the thyroid affects so many bodily actions. When the GAPS diet was introduced, the lady in question didn't know whether it would work or what benefits there would be to using this diet, but she was concerned enough about her welfare to want to do something to positively enhance the lifestyle that she found was being limited by the symptoms listed here. These will differ from patient to patient, so don't look out for things that you don't suffer from. Simply make a list of your symptoms so you can follow your progress through the introduction of the diet through to the conclusion that the diet is working for you.

Dizziness and Palpitations

Common to many sufferers, the patient was concerned about the way that her brain seemed to be reacting when she got out of bed or when she rolled over in the night. These weren't just coincidental. She knew that they were symptoms of a larger ailment.

Dysfunction of Cognitive Processes

This does not happen to all patients, but this particular patient was finding that logical reasoning and thought processes were difficult to keep in check. When she was talking sometimes, she would lose the conversation midstream and this worried her.

Asthma

Perhaps not Hashimoto related but worthwhile mentioning because the GAPS DIET helped with this. The patient was taking her medications at regular intervals before the GAPS diet was introduced.

Problems with Digestion

This is an extremely common symptom associated with Hashimoto disease and the patient found that it was hard to digest meat in particular and that she suffered from GERD after eating anything at all and had problems lying down at night. Many sufferers of acid reflux are tempted by the medications that they can buy over the counter to treat it, rather than facing the fact that these are actually contributing to the overall problems. They can cause constipation, which can in turn cause all the problems associated with over-fermentation because the food stays in the stomach for too long a time without going through the normal processes one would expect. People who suffer from constipation also resort to taking medications on a regular basis and if you read the instructions on medications of this nature, they always give a warning that they should not be used on a regular basis because they encourage the gut or the colon to become lazy, thus making long term problems even worse than they originally were.

Changes in blood sugar levels

The patient noticed this from blood tests and what it caused was triggering bouts of energy followed by bouts of lethargy. There was no consistency to her life because of this and people around her were unsure of what mood she would have upon approach. That was making her social life and life with the family difficult.

Eye problems

I remember a fellow sufferer of Hashimoto's disease explaining that eye problems could be associated with Hashimoto's and this patient also found that. In fact, it's more common than you may imagine. The placement of the pituitary gland could be one of the reasons and since this works in conjunction with the thyroid, if the thyroid is off, then chances are that pain will happen in this area behind the eye.

Insomnia and weight gain

These are very common among sufferers of Hashimoto's disease and patients may resort to taking drugs to help them to sleep. In fact, doing this may be considered a cop out because learning relaxation techniques and being on the correct diet will help this on its own. However, tell that to someone who hasn't slept well for as long as she can remember and it takes a while to put all the symptoms together and to realize that they are associated.

Introducing the GAPS diet

The patient introduced the GAPS diet and stayed on it for a year. During this time, she learned which foods were tolerable and which were not. This is a diet that was produced by Dr. Natasha Campbell-McBride. Belonging to the British Society for Environmental Medicine and having a background in neurology, who better to come up with a diet that deals with autoimmune illnesses and that helps people to cope through changing what they eat? If you are not convinced, then read on because the results that the patient got from going on this diet were astounding and others have acclaimed this diet as a wonderful eye opener and one that has changed their lives forever. GAPS stands for Gut and Psychology syndrome and her book outlining the diet gives clear and concise instructions for users to follow. There have been several people that have written guides but to my knowledge this is the first one that relates solely to the connection between the GAPS diet and Hashimoto's. What the diet does is retrain your way of thinking, so that you can replace foods that are harmful to you but which are now common parts of your diet with foods that are tastier and that are not harmful.

It may be worthwhile watching this doctor who trained in traditional medicine giving a talk on the diet if you are considering it because she is inspirational and if her YouTube video does not persuade you, perhaps the results of our patient will. In the video on YouTube she explains in a very simple and easy to understand way that we are making ourselves ill by the foods that we choose to eat. You may have ideas as to which foods are healthy ones and which are not but you need to bear in mind that you are highly influenced by advertisements and what you see as positive may actually be damaging to your gut. Leaky gut happens when the cells that line the gut are not reproducing as they should and protecting the rest of the body from toxins. As these cells have a limited lifespan, it's essential that they do regenerate but the foods that you are eating may not be allowing this, and what this means in simple terms is that your stomach lining is insufficiently strong to stop bacteria passing into the body. That's bad news.

The lady patient that we were discussing who has been on the GAPS diet for a year found the following results:

Inflammation

Almost all inflammation in her body ceased and although from time to time there is inflammation, this has been limited to such an extent that she no longer suffers brain fog, or lack of being able to think clearly.

Asthma drugs – Weaned off these entirely and does not need them anymore.

Digestive Problems

Completely cured! And that's huge because these included all kinds of uncomfortable ailments. All gone.

Eye Pain

While she still had floaters from time to time, there was absolutely no pain any more.

Insomnia – gone and now gets a good night's sleep without any kind of medication.

Weight gain

Stopped in its tracks. The patient has a stable weight and much more control over her size.

Thyroid function

Vastly improved since introducing this diet, and avoiding Lactose.

The doctor who came up with this diet says that people should realize the impact of the gut on all health issues because this is a huge percentage of the organic matter that makes up a human being. Ignore it, and you allow illness to happen. That's why the GAPS diet is considered so important in the fight against Hashimoto's disease.

We felt that this explanation was necessary before telling you more about the GAPS diet because those who know the significance of the diet are much more likely to try harder. No one actually enjoys being in bad health and the GAPS diet helps you to restore the balance of your health to an optimum level. By replacing foods that are known to irritate the action of the cells within the gut, you give your gut a chance to replenish its lining and thus protect the body from invasion by toxins. Think of the size of the gut. Think of the amount of risk because the doctor who came up with the GAPS diet has been working with women and children for a very long time and does know what she is talking about. She isn't approaching this from a commercial viewpoint in order to make money. She is approaching it from scientifically based and proven information.

I cannot emphasize enough that the GAPS diet helps you to address any health problems that you have and put your body back on track. She has dealt with fussy eaters, she has dealt with people addicted to sweet foods, the lactose intolerant and any other person who has gone to her with health problems which they believe may have their origins in the gut and the success rate of her work is super impressive. For your Hashimoto's this is a real way of dealing with the gut problems that are allowing the sluggishness of the T4 to T3 conversion and that's key to helping your thyroid restore its natural balance.

Getting Ready to Take on the Challenge of a New Diet

The problem that surrounds everyone when they try a new diet is the temptation to eat foods that are not permitted. People who are slimming often do this since the temptation is too great. All around them, they have the availability of foods that will tempt them and the shops are filled with them. Not only that, but relatives will also tempt them. It's not that they don't care. It's just that they are trying to be encouraging and don't know the harm that they are doing.

Thus in order to prepare yourself for this diet, you need to approach it in a much different way. This time, it's not just so that you can be slim. It's going to put years of good health ahead of you instead of suffering, so if you have a family who are not going to follow the same diet as you, you need to sit down and explain why it is that you are going to try to make this diet a way of life. One of the ways of explaining is that food is fuel. Basically what you put into your body will determine how good your health will be. If you decided to put diesel into a car that needed gas, it wouldn't work. Your body isn't working because normal diet is actually destroying you and making you feel worse. The reason why this explanation is necessary is that loved ones want the best for you and if they know that your health is at stake are less likely to try and tempt you to eat unhealthy choices.

You need to prepare your kitchen, so that the food that you have for your own diet is strictly within the parameters of the diet chosen. If you can encourage others in the family to eat the same foods that you choose to eat, all well and good, but if they are young and in good health, they may not feel inclined to do that. Food preparation has to be a very disciplined thing. If you have to prepare food that does not fall within your diet, it can be very tempting to help yourself when no one is looking. You have to draw a line and know where your limitations are. It may sound harsh, but think of food in the same way as you think of medicines and it becomes easier. If you were to mess around with your medicines and take them when you felt like it, they wouldn't work. The diet is like that too. If you decide to change your eating habits, you need sufficient discipline to be able to do it. If you attempt half-heartedly, it won't work. We have given you a choice in this book of several diets and we have also explained all about FODMAP foods as this is very relevant indeed. You may think that the diet that you are on is good, but labels are often deceptive and you may, by now, have learned that high FODMAP foods are not always obvious.

Thus, you need to make a note so that you can see which foods are acceptable and which are not. Keep a separate place in the larder so that your foods are clearly marked and you can use the right ingredients without worrying about whether you've included something that is forbidden. I would suggest that you make a note of the foods that are permitted and learn this by heart, so that when you go shopping, you know exactly what you are looking for. People who stay on the Paleo or GAPS diet say that it's a little hard to start off with but that they soon learn permitted and non-permitted foods.

One thing that dieters find hard is that snacks get in the way of progress and you are going to find that this is the case even when you are dieting for health purposes. Thus, you need to decide which foods you can consider as your luxury snacks. For example, making cookies on the Paleo diet from permitted foods gives you an extra choice, just as choosing foods on the GAP diet as luxury foods allows you to snack without the worry of actually breaking the diet. You just have to switch your mind set, so that you see foods in a different light.

It takes a while to get accustomed to a new diet. If you think that it will help you, there's nothing to stop you from going on an intermittent fast before you start your new diet. I would suggest that you decide at which hour you will start this, and during this fasting time, you are giving your body a chance to catch up and get rid of all that bad food. Drinking water or nettle tea during this period will help you to eliminate all the bad foods which are in your digestive tract before you start your new diet and that gives you an added bit of incentive to be enthusiastic about the new diet that you know is going to help your health.

Stocking up on the right things

One of the things you will need for the GAPS diet is bone broth and chicken broth because you are going to need it. Make sure that you have plenty because this really acts as a great help when you are preparing food.

Another thing you can prepare in advance are things like Squash and if you bake this in advance and freeze it, it's really useful as a part of the diet.

You may not think about it, but if you can visit a farm shop and get really fresh meat that is grass fed, stocking up on this is a wise idea too. You won't be tempted to pop down to the supermarket at the last minute when you need meat. You can save yourself an awful lot of hassle if you freeze meat already prepared into meal sized portions because this saves so much preparation and the prep time that you take is the most likely time that you will cheat on your diet, whereas if you have things prepared, you are more likely to keep to the diet.

Make sure that you have plenty of fermented foods like sauerkraut because you need to change the way you look at foods like this and include plenty within your diet to protect the lining of your stomach. You will also need loads of fresh vegetables and bulk buying is a great idea, plus learning to store in a dry place that won't be affected by heat.

Make a whole load of vegetables soups because these will be handy and if you make things in advance when you have more time, you are more likely to stick to the diet.

Meal plan. This is vital to success. If you meal plan, you can work out which foods to prepare in advance on days when you are at home and that way, you won't have to be looking around for different ingredients on workdays when you don't have the mental energy to cope with it.

When planning to go onto the Paleo diet, it's also a very good idea to detox before you start and here, I would suggest that you go on an intermittent fast before you start. The problem is that the diet can be a bit of a shock to the system and if you detox between your normal diet and the Paleo diet, this helps considerably to break that shock so that your body is satisfied with the foods that you introduce. I would suggest that you do this from 8 in the evening until the next day and that in this time, you drink mint tea or nettle tea and lots of water and then start the diet with a great breakfast of salmon and poached egg because this is relatively filling and satisfying and will make you feel sated.

Again, with this diet, you need to remember that preparation in advance saves heartbreak, and if you use weekends to prepare food for the week in batches, this is probably the easier way of handing the change in your diet. You are going to find that paleo foods are more expensive. For example, pasture fed meat will be more expensive as will vegetables that are grown in an ecological way. They always are more expensive, so you need to have a budget set for what you can afford and work out recipes that don't use up that budget too quickly. If you do, you may be tempted to stop because you find the Paleo diet too expensive to continue. It doesn't have to be if you space your meals and work out a sensible diet for the week.

There are things that you will never have heard of that you need to stock up on such as Coconut Aminos and it may be worthwhile knowing that coconut aminos can be bought online at health websites or websites such as Amazon and you really do need to keep these in stock.

Another thing you need to invest in ready for the diets is Tupper ware and freezer bags with plenty of labels so that you can manage your food better and keep everything fresh. Believe me, you will get through loads of Tupper ware because you will be storing things like your grandmother used to and that means that you always have something on hand if snacking cravings come on and that's important.

Your preparation is vital. So many people have started with good intentions only to find that they fall apart after a few days because they run out of something or because there's nothing immediately available to tuck into that falls within the diet that they are on. Thus, meal planning, having a day cooking a week, and making sure that you have the entire ingredient you need is vital to success.

Without this preparation, chances are that you will fail when you try to go onto one of these diets. You do need to familiarize yourself with all the ins and outs of the diet and be really prepared, so it's better to put it off for a week and give yourself a chance to prepare than to start half-heartedly, thinking that you can stock up on supplies later. It doesn't really work like that. You need to keep yourself stocked up and have things available that are allowed. That way, you don't have the same level of temptation to come off the diet at a whim.

Be aware of the foods that you will have to avoid at all costs. In fact, if you have a way of keeping these out of your larder do so because that will take away the temptation. For example, on the Paleo diet, avoid the following:

- Potatoes – too starchy
- Coffee in all formats

- Chickpeas
- Quinoa – Lean meat is much better for you

Have a list of no no foods and make sure that you don't have them there to tempt you. If these are foods that the rest of the family eats, suggest keeping them in a locked cupboard so that the temptation is taken away. Unfortunately, even though you may be starting with the best of intentions, you may easily be tempted if you have these available to you. Carry around a bottle of water so that when you are visiting friends for a coffee, you can simply choose your water and not feel left out.

Look at the recipe range available

This is something that can get you interested in your diet and if you use sites such as Pinterest, you will find that you are not as limited as you first thought. However, don't cook too many dishes that cost you too much or you will give up – thinking that you cannot afford to stay on the diet and use money as the excuse. This isn't actually true. You can diet on the Paleo and GAPS diets without spending an absolute fortune. You just have to learn to plan your menus so that you don't come across a situation where cost gets in the way.

The biggest thing to remember when you are changing over to a new diet is that it's going to be hard to start off with and if you are unprepared, you are likely to back out of the diet and cheat. However, if you do meal planning ahead of time and have a freezer load of food already prepared, you don't have the same excuse.

I would suggest that you start your preparation weeks before you actually change the diet. This means that the food that you have already prepared gives you your staple diet and as you buy more food, you can prepare and put meals away for the future. Learn to cook in batches as this is a much more efficient way to cook, especially if you have a freezer. Learn to bottle foods and this will help you because it means that you have a steady supply of foods. Learn to store vegetables so that you don't waste them.

One of the best methods for storing vegetables is in a very dry place, wrapped in newspaper. However, if these are vegetables that you can prepare into broth, do so in advance and split everything up into meal sized portions. It will make the whole procedure of being on a diet much easier if you don't suddenly have to produce something independent from what the rest of the family are eating. That can be a real put down and may spell the end of your diet that is bad news. Thus, preparation is everything and having a great variety of foods and ready prepared meals means that the food you will prepare will be just like convenience foods from the point of view that you just have to heat them but they will be a lot more nutritious.

Get used to using herbs because there are some wonderful flavors that you can add to make your broths taste so much better. If you are going to use parsnips, these are wonderful in a broth but imagine what you add by using the right herbs and spices. Get excited about recipes before you actually go onto the diet and have many meals prepared in advance to ensure your success.

I have seen people who have successfully kept to their diet because they prepared while others were too tempted to fail because they didn't have the food available readily and that's a huge mistake to make. If you find that you have to prepare one meal for family members and another for you, having all the meals ready prepared makes this a lot less painful and easy! Believe me, I have been cooking for people with varying diets for most of my life and pre-prepared food is the exact reason why people choose convenience foods. It makes their lives easier. Working on this premise, it makes sense that if you have a baking or cooking day once a week and refill the freezer for the week, you will find yourself much more likely to get into the routine of the diet and stick to it.

Healing Hashimoto's Thyroiditis With The GAPS Diet

When it comes to healing your gut in order to deal with Hashimoto's, you first need to figure out what is causing the problem. These could include food intolerances, stress, infections etc. Once you know what is causing the problem, the next step is to get rid of the triggers and finally restore your gut health as well as gut barrier in order to deal with a leaky gut problem. This is where the GAPS diet comes in.

GAPS stands for Gut and Psychology syndrome. This diet mainly focuses on introduction of high amounts of fats, proteins (from nuts, seeds, fish and meat), unprocessed fruits, probiotics, and non-starchy vegetables. It also eliminates foods like complex carbohydrates, starch and all processed foods. The diet especially focuses on cutting out refined sugars and starch since they feed pathogens in your body. So, getting rid of the sugars also means getting rid of pathogens. This diet has been recognized worldwide to cure autoimmune disorders by healing the gut. Thus, it's important to eliminate those foods from your larder that are warned against.

Adopting the GAPS diet can prove to be hard

for you since there are lots of foods you love that you will have to give up. You should just try to focus on what you are able to eat and not what you are unable to eat. You should also know that you would not have to give up on all the foods you love since there are substitutes available. Try to have the right foods at all time (stock them up) to avoid any kind of temptation and keep away the foods you should avoid. As we stated in the preparation chapter, you need to think of the new foods as being prepared and ready just like convenience foods would be. Therefore, if you cook up meals in advance, you are less likely to stray from the diet and will be happy even on working days to follow the diet as planned.

You should also know that everyone is different and what works for you might not work for others and vice versa. You might be intolerant to a certain product like milk, which means it will not be in your diet and may be present in others. The extent of the thyroiditis can also determine what will and what will not work. Besides, everyone's immune system is different so they all work differently. You must first get tested in order to know what will work best for you.

Effective Techniques to Shed Your Hashimoto

Weight

One of the most common complaints of those suffering from Hashimoto's is the difficulty that they face when it comes to losing weight. If you're suffering from this aspect, then you have come to the right place. The following chapters will show you how you can change the metabolism and how this in turn will help your gut health and help you to change your metabolism rate.

Healing Hashimoto's Thyroiditis with the GAPS Diet

When it comes to healing your gut in order to deal with Hashimoto's, you first need to figure out what is causing the problem. These could include food intolerances, stress, infections etc. Once you know what is causing the problem, the next step is to get rid of the triggers and finally restore your gut health as well as gut barrier in order to deal with a leaky gut problem. This is where the GAPS diet comes in. You can usually tell if it's food intolerance by cutting out foods and then introducing them again. Doctors that specialize in allergies and what this means is eating one food at a time and then gradually introducing other foods have used the

Stone Age diet for this. It takes a bit of time to do but it can help you to see logically which foods are causing you problems and whether the GAPS diet or the PALEO diet is the right choice in your particular case.

GAPS stands for Gut and Psychology syndrome. This diet mainly focuses on introduction of high amounts of fats, proteins (from nuts, seeds, fish and meat), unprocessed fruits, probiotics, and non-starchy vegetables. It also eliminates foods like complex carbohydrates, starch and all processed foods. The diet especially focuses on cutting out refined sugars and starch since they feed pathogens in your body. So, getting rid of the sugars also means getting rid of pathogens. This diet has been recognized worldwide to cure autoimmune disorders by healing the gut. In fact, if you are unconvinced do watch the video on YouTube on the GAPS diet which is given by the doctor who was previously mentioned in this book because it's very convincing and may be all it takes to make you see that your health really is in your own hands.

Adopting the GAPS diet can prove to be hard for you since there are lots of foods you love that you will have to give up. You should just try to focus on what you are able to eat and not what you are unable to eat. You should also know that you will not have to give up on all the foods you love since there are substitutes available. Try to have the right foods at all time (stock them up) to avoid any kind of temptation and keep away the foods you should avoid. Although that sounds easy, you also need to take account of social gatherings when food will be provided that doesn't fall within your diet. If you can take foods with you, this stops embarrassment and means that you can stay on your diet and your friends will understand if you explain that this is for health reasons, rather than being a fad diet.

You should also know that everyone is different and what works for you might not work for others and vice versa. You might be intolerant to a certain product like milk, which means it will not be in your diet and may be present in others. The extent of the thyroiditis can also determine what will and what will not work. Besides, everyone's immune system is different so they all work differently. You must first get tested in order to know what will work best for you.

The tests that are available to the public on food intolerances vary considerably and you would be well advised to visit your doctor and find out what is available to you in your hometown. There are some testing facilities that charge expensively for these tests, though others may deal with them by looking to see what your allergies are and this is done by a series of skin pricks which show up as red if there is a food intolerance. Since this is being done purely to help you assess which diet to go on, your doctor can advise on which is the best method but you need to explain to him that you are having a lot of gut problems and want to cut down on those foods that you really think may be causing it. Your doctor will also know your medical history so is very likely to already know the problems that you are encountering, so is the best person to ask about testing.

(h) Effective Techniques to Shed Your Hashimoto Weight

One of the most common complaints of those suffering from Hashimoto's is the difficulty that they face when it comes to losing weight. If you're suffering from Hashimoto's thyroiditis, then you must be taking a certain kind of medication as well. For those who take a replacement hormone, losing weight appears to be a bigger challenge as compared to those not taking the replacement hormone. Are you tired of waiting around for a miracle to happen while you eat healthy and exercise as well? Do you feel as if nothing can help you achieve your dream weight? Here are a few secrets to weight loss according to the latest research. However, before applying these strategies, make sure to get your hormones in balance as much as you can.

(i) Stop Considering the Outdated Metabolism Model

For a Hashimoto's patient, the old model of energy in versus energy out isn't the solution to the puzzle. We saw a lot of Hashimoto's patients who were unable to lose weight even while they were on calorie reduction all the time. It doesn't work because the gut is not acting in the normal way. You can't expect to diet when your metabolism dictates how fast those calories are burnt. Metabolism that is out of synch is the reason that you can't lose weight, rather than what you are eating. Thus, dieting isn't the answer. Changing your diet is, as this will help to correct the metabolism and help you to become like those people who lose weight more easily.

135

While it is still important to keep a moderately negative energy balance, there are other factors in your nutrition that may interact with your hormones.

Your body doesn't work like a machine; it has a lot of mechanisms to control your metabolism.

(j)   Immune System as a Big Factor

Research has proven that your immune system is actually a huge issue when it comes to losing weight. Dr. Datis who is known as the leading expert on thyroid treatment, and the issues relating to its functionality and the medicine carried out a recent seminar. He has managed to offer an effective treatment using functional medicine, which is referred to as the Neuroendocrine Immunology of Exercise. He explained the new findings of this latest research in this seminar as well. According to him, an entirely new model has been developed to study the reasons behind the tendency of patients leaning toward weight gain.

The new model clearly talks about different plausible causes of weight issues which are directly or indirectly associated with your immune system. The model makes more sense when dealing with people with Hashimoto's, because it's a disease of an autoimmune nature and links with the thyroid hormones.

Are you tired of waiting around for a miracle to happen while you eat healthy and exercise as well? Do you feel as if nothing can help you achieve your dream weight? Here are a few secrets to weight loss according to the latest research. However, before applying these strategies, make sure to get your hormones in balance as much as you can.

Dr Kharrazian states that the new immune system indicates a total of four reasons when it comes to stubborn weight gain. Here are four reasons that associate your weight gain with the immune system:

- The presence of a mix of bacteria in your stomach/gut.
- A leaky gut is also responsible for the stubbornness that is known as intestinal permeability.
- Inflammation of low-grade intensity.
- Dietary proteins which are immune

reactive.

You must consider your body as an ecosystem, or better yet think of it as an interconnected series of ecosystems. Your digestive tract is in fact the most complex one among all of these. It is also among the most dynamic ones. Each individual has their own personal bacteria mix, along with other such organisms that reside in their stomachs. The kind of mix you receive is actually determined by your own unique genetic profile, along with the kind of diets you consume and the medications that you choose to take. Moreover, the environment has a strong impact on the genetic profile as well.

On an average, your body consists of about a hundred trillion various kinds of cells and more than a thousand various species of bacteria as well. A vast majority of ninety percent of the bacteria species is from two families by the name of Firmicutes and Bacteriodetes.

The essential thing for you to remember is that a certain kind of balance of bacteria will make your body experience a reduced ability to lose weight. The research of the modern era has clearly shown that a balance of these two aforementioned bacterial species matters a lot in determining whether you are able to shed weight or not. When we take overweight people into consideration, their bodies generally consist of more Firmicutes bacteria as compared to the Bacteriodetes.

The balance of these two species of bacteria has the ability to generate signals of a certain kind, which inform the genes in your intestines responsible for producing fat cells. The most common species of bacteria found in probiotics, Lactobacillus bacteria, actually increases your weight. This basically means that although the probiotics are highly beneficial when it comes to your gut's ecosystems, these are not helpful in aiding the shedding of weight. That's not actually what they are designed for. They are designed to help digestion.

By simply increasing the Bacteriodetes, you can actually lose weight as well. The Firmicutes are actually quite fond of junk food and in order to feed for the increasing of your weight, you can simply eat similarly to an average American. But in order to starve these bacteria, which will help you lose weight, you can consider a change.

Apparently these bacteria are quite fond of plants.

So essentially, the best possible way to increase the overall number of these bacteria is to amplify your consumption of plant based edibles and fiber. Get your vegetables. Food quality matters and if you eat foods that are untreated by pesticides and chemicals, then this helps considerably.

Fix your Gut first

Most people suffering from Hashimoto's tend to suffer from issues such as a leaky gut syndrome or intestinal permeability. According to new research, this also leads to an increase of fat content around your organs. In the case of leaky gut, your intestines basically lose the innate ability to prevent tiny particles of all kinds from entering your internal blood stream. According to the latest research, a connection can be formed between the breakdown process of your gut barrier system and a fatty liver.

As was explained in the video by the inventor of the GAPS diet, what happens to the digestive system is that the lining is replaced within a relatively short space of time, but if you don't eat the right foods, this doesn't happen and this results in leaky gut.

Moreover, zonulin is a protein that leaks in to

your bloodstream when this barrier experiences a breakdown. The intestines for binding of the junctions essentially use the protein. This is increased when a person becomes obese. Lipopolysaccharides are toxins that are a result of bacteria production, and these are also associated with obesity and diabetes. So the bottom line is if you're looking to get a smaller gut, then you must ensure the healing of your leaky gut. A good method of achieving this is altering your diet, as we'll discuss in the second book of this series, and supplement with a dose of 20g L-Glutamine daily to help you to achieve this.

Get rid of Inflammation

Inflammation is a common sign of an autoimmune disease. New research is showing that obesity can also be regarded as a kind of inflammatory condition. One thing that is quite certain is that the fat tissue known as the adipose tissue causes the production of inflammation in the body on its own. This leads to the initiation of a rather destructive cycle of abnormal gut bacteria along with a leaky gut, which again leads to a process of resistance for insulin and leptin. If you take a long time to digest food or you do not go to the toilet regularly, this may even make the situation much worse.

This in turn makes the glucose unable to enter the cells of your body. When a case of such happens where the body's glucose is unable to enter the cells, then it starts to convert into fat in your liver. These are the fat cells that restart this entire process all over again.

Leptin is among the primary hormones that take part in processes of hunger and metabolism along with control when it comes to storage of your fats and carbohydrates. The word Leptin, by the way, is derived from the Greek word "leptos," which literally translates as thin. The quantity of Leptin production in your body is directly linked with your weight loss and gain. The resistance of Leptin is actually quite similar to that of insulin. In the resistance of insulin, the elevated insulin levels tend to make the fat cells even more resistant to insulin's activity, and the same goes for leptin.

When the body experiences chronically elevated leptin levels, then you end up eating a lot more than what you're supposed to, as your body makes you do so. The abnormal bacteria in your gut along with a leaky gut also feed this process.

To get rid of inflammation, you need to eat diet rich in Omega3, Vitamin D, Gut Irritants, and immune reactive proteins. We will discuss the entire dietary plan in the next book of this series. All you need to know at this moment is that you are going to say goodbye to processed food and say hello to a paleo diet in order to get rid of it i.e., inflammation. But one more thing that you need to know is that there are proteins that you must avoid, because these certain kinds of protein have the ability to enhance the inflammation. Every other living thing on this planet is made of proteins. When your body experiences an autoimmune disease, then that makes your immune system undergo confusion between your personal proteins and that of a foreign body such as an allergic food or a virus. There are those proteins as well which have the ability to trigger an immune response, and this can lead to inflammation. Such proteins can be found in dairy, soy, and gluten, along with other foods that are called cross reactors.

You are required to eliminate these proteins from your diet if you wish to lose weight, as this will ensure the unwinding of the cycle of inflammation. This will help you to stop the weight gain by treating the root cause.

Causes of Hashimoto's and the Foods to be Avoided During Hashimoto's

There are many things that we consume on a daily basis that could have triggered this disease, but like they say "It is never too late." You can still consider all the precautionary measures in order to support your body in fighting against Hashimoto's. Diet itself is controlled and connected by other factors like exercise, spiritual therapy, and mental therapy. Anyway, let's start with a quick view of all the foods that contain the ingredients to make the recipe of Hashimoto's on the inside of your body.

Gluten

It has been established that there is a very close relationship between gluten and Hashimoto's, such that if you are found to have Hashimoto's, you are often tested for gluten intolerance. So, what is gluten? Gluten is a composite protein of gliadin and glutenin. Gliadin's molecular structure resembles that of the thyroid gland. So, when you take food rich in gluten, the gliadin is likely to breach the gut's protective barrier and then enter the bloodstream. This is referred to as leaky gut. When the gliadin enters the bloodstream, the immune system releases antibodies to destroy this foreign body. Since gliadin is very similar to the thyroid in terms of molecular structure, the same antibodies that destroy the gliadin also start attacking the thyroid. Therefore, if you already have Hashimoto's or any other autoimmune thyroid disease, you need to stay away from gluten. As such, you ought to embrace a gluten-free diet because this kind of reaction and destruction of the thyroid gland can even last up to six months. Adopting a gluten free diet "occasionally" won't be enough; you need to ensure that your diet is 100% gluten free to prevent any autoimmune destruction of the thyroid.

Why is that a problem? The trouble is that foods are not always labeled correctly and that people don't actually read labels. You do need to take care with this if you have a gluten intolerance because it can hide in all kinds of foods. The first things that you need to look for on the label are Barley, Rye and wheat. That means that things such as cereals, breads, cakes and biscuits are the main culprits but they are not the only ones.

Processed foods can contain gluten and so can the following foods, so you need to be really careful about your choices of foods:

Pasta, salad dressings, sausages, sauces and seasonings, crackers and cookies, cereals, breads, bread crumb coatings, broths and soups, etc.

There are so many that it's difficult to list all of them, but you can see by the diversity of things that gluten is contained in that you really do need to take care. Did you know that licking an envelope or the back of a stamp could also cause a gluten reaction? It can in some countries, so be very aware of everything that you take into your mouth.

Dairy Products

Milk-based products have a host of proteins that can also cause immune reactions. These include casein casomorphin—a protein that closely resembles morphine—whey, and milk butyrophilin. These proteins are known as "cross-reactors" because they closely resemble gluten proteins, and can cause similar immune responses in the body. To avoid this situation, you need to avoid the entire list of dairy products given below that are ultimately made from milk.

- Butter.
- Cheeses.
- Cow milk.
- Creams.
- Frozen desserts.
- Goat milk.
- Margarine.
- Mayonnaise.
- Sheep milk.
- Yogurt.

Sugar and Caffeine-Containing Food

The decision on whether to incorporate sugar and caffeine-containing food basically depends upon your level of hypothyroidism and your level of adrenal fatigue. For the most part, it is simply not advisable to eat food that contains sugar or caffeine. Sugar and caffeine both can up the ante on the overproduction of hormones that cause stress—named as cortisol and adrenaline—and the fact that they both hinder the thyroid function makes them an enemy for the people who have Hashimoto's. It's also known that spikes in blood sugar will result in low-level inflammation, which is something you should be trying to avoid when suffering from

Hashimoto's. This is another reason why sweeteners should not be used. These may imitate sugar, but they also imitate the spikes and this can be harmful to the thyroid. The trouble with sweeteners is that many contain chemicals that are harmful to the body after prolonged use, and as they are sweeter than sugar and the duration of the sugar spike is less, you tend to need more of them to compensate for the sugar spike being short lived. Avoid them if at all possible.

Goitrogens Containing Food

Goitrogens interfere in the working of the endocrine system that produces hormones for the thyroid glands. When thyroids in your body get deprived of the hormone they must have to work efficiently, they ultimately swell. This swelling for you springs out another disease called Goiter, and where you were just dealing with one disease, now you have two. Thus, after your professional doctor's recommendations, you have to pick out all those food products that you deem might help you come out from this horrifying disease. Now, here is a limited list for your information so that you can see the kind of foods that need to be avoided. For further safety measures, you need to be more careful of all the food that you deem might have even a slight trace of goitrogens. All the goitrogens containing food are listed below:

- Broccoli.
- Kohlrabi.
- Cauliflower.
- Rutabaga.
- Brussels sprouts.
- Kale.
- Cabbage.

Cook Away Your Goitrogens

Now here is the deal. If it gets really difficult for you to find food that does NOT contain goitrogens in it, then you need not worry yourself about that. What you should do is to cook those goitrogen-containing foods before consuming them, and it will be just fine for you since cooking kills all the effects it could produce when not cooked. Thus think of these vegetables in reasonable quantities and thoroughly cooked at all times and avoid things like coleslaw or uncooked vegetables if you want to avoid a goiter being formed in your thyroid area.

Soy

Many people would recommend that you not use soy at all. Well, it could be harmful unless it is eaten in moderation. Tempeh, for example, could be used without any fear of harming your body. Some of the forms of fermented soy include tempeh (as mentioned above), natto, tamari, shoyu, and miso. This type of soy does not block protein digestion and also, it is not a menace to your thyroids. However, the unfermented soy would be harmful, since it has the capacity to stop the process of protein digestion, and also the enlargement of goiter since it contains goitrogens.

Here is a list of unfermented soy products that could be harmful to your condition because of the potential altering of your hormonal profile and the containment of goitrogens:

- Soymilk.
- Soy Tofu.
- Soy Ice Cream.
- Soy nuts.
-

Soy has also been linked to cancers such as breast cancer, so it is best to avoid these in any great quantity.

Seeds, Grain, Nuts, and Other Cross Reactors

So, as discussed above, other than soy and goitrogen-containing food items, what else one must avoid using are seeds, grains (Gluten!), nuts, nightshades, alcohol, dairy, eggs, and legumes. This might seem like a hard nut to crack, but once you get to know about all other delicious dishes that you can have during Hashimoto's, it will not look like such a gigantic challenge. The reason why these foods should be cut from our diet is that nuts are one of the top allergens and most common food sensitivities. People with autoimmune disease are most likely to have a leaky gut, which ultimately increases their susceptibility to developing food allergies and food sensitivities. This means that people with an autoimmune disease such as Hashimoto's are more likely to have a sensitivity or allergy to nuts, grains, and seeds than other people. Therefore, it is better if one avoids using them.

Here is a list of grains that you'll need to eliminate from your diet:

- Amaranth.

- Barley.
- Buckwheat.
- Bulgur.
- Corn.
- Couscous.
- Kamut.
- Millet.
- Oats.
- Quinoa.
- Rice.
- Rye.
- Spelt.
- Wheat.
- Wheat germ.

Mercury-Containing Diet

The newest studies also demonstrate that heavy metal exposure can trigger autoimmune attacks. Especially the excessive intake of mercury could potentially cause Hashimoto's. Here's a question that might tell you what caused the level of mercury higher than its limit in your body: do you love eating fish or seafood? Because fish can contain a large amount of mercury. You might need to hold your desire of consuming fish in big portions and always aim for fish that is low in terms of mercury contamination.

These fish include Butterfish, Herring, Mullet, Shrimp, Tilapia, Hake, and Whitefish.

On the other hand you should expect high levels of mercury in Mackerel, Marlin, Swordfish, Tilefish and Tuna.

Other than that, you find mercury in dental amalgams as well.

Fluoride-Containing Diet

Fluoride is another common chemical that can further aggravate your condition. It would be surprising for you to know how many things that you use every day in your life that comprise within them traces of fluoride. The list includes water and toothpaste.

You may not be aware of it, but if your water supply comes from a deep well, chances are that the fluoride content is high. Other notable items that hide fluoride are teas and processed foods. As far as fluoride is concerned, you need to think about the amount of treatment that water has in your country and then about the amount of processing that the food goes through on its way to the consumer. If you have a highly processed item, then it's likely to have more fluoride in it. That's why freshness is paramount.

Toxins and Xenoestrogens-Containing Diet

Xenoestrogens are the most powerful endocrine disruptors, which means that all the hormones that are under the supervision of the endocrine system get seriously disturbed and, eventually, the balance of hormones becomes imbalanced.

Likewise, all those substances that mimic the body's estrogen present in pesticides, fertilizers, body care products, plastics, etc., are all themselves the toxins which are used by us in daily life. We never know that the air we breathe and the water we consume all contain traces of these elements that are disturbing our endocrine system, breaking down the function of immune system and thus, potentially causing Hashimoto's. So how can you avoid this? You can introduce HEPA filters in the home and use air filters that help you to keep the air fresh within your home. Using an ionizer may prove useful as well.

Step 1: Getting Rid of Food Intolerances

Let us now begin with the first step of the GAPS diet, which entails the removal of food intolerances. The foods you should avoid eating are based on your body's adrenalin fatigue and your level of hypothyroidism. But often, it is always advisable to stay away from caffeine and sugar since they can lead to the over production of stress hormones cortisol and adrenalin. Here is an overview of the foods you should avoid:

Food you have found out to be intolerant to. Some of the common foods are gluten, dairy, soy, nightshades (peppers, tomatoes, potatoes, and eggplants), corn, eggs, and fructose.

All sweeteners and sugar- you should only take honey but in small amounts

Any vegetable that is starchy- these are like yams, cassava, sweet potatoes, Jerusalem artichoke, and potatoes

Any type of soy- soy milk, tofu, soy protein, tempeh, tofu and others

Lectins, which are a major cause for leaky gut- you should avoid beans (except white beans and Lima), peanut butter, nuts unless they are soaked, peanut oil, and the other lectins

All highly refined foods

All grains- oats, buckwheat, quinoa, wheat, rice, barley, and corn etc.

If you have hypothyroidism, avoid all foods that suppress the thyroid. These are all the cruciferous vegetables like broccoli, spinach, cabbage, kales, soy, Brussels sprouts and turnips

Fruits that are high in the glycemic index- these are mangoes, raisins, canned fruits, watermelons, pineapple, grapes and dried fruits

You should also not consume any kind of alcohol

Coffee- as hard as it may be, coffee should be

avoided. Most of the people who have gluten sensitivity react to coffee as if it is some sort of gluten. Avoid it so that you can be sure that it won't be an immune trigger.

You should also avoid canned foods

Agave syrup- avoid it since its main carbohydrate is a fructose (it's in complex form)

Algae- should be avoided because it can further aggravate your immune system, which is already disturbed

Apple juice and balsamic vinegar- this is because it has sugar added to it when it is being processed

Amaranth and arrowroot- they are loaded with starches

Aloe Vera- should only be taken if your digestive issues subside

Baking powder and all kinds of raising agents

You should avoid pollen at all costs since it really irritates an already damaged gut

Burdock root because it contains mucilage and FOS

Cheeses, processed cheeses, and cheese spreads

You should not chew gum also since it contains either sugar or sugar substitutes

Don't take cocoa powder also unless it is raw and there are no sugars added

Corn syrups

Milk from any animal, coconut milk, rice and soy

Commercial ketchup and ice cream

Fish- either smoked, breaded, preserved or canned with sauces

All pasta

This is a very comprehensive list and while some people may be intolerant to the above mentioned foods, you may not. Therefore, I would advise you to get rid of all the above foods then start incorporating the foods one by one as in the Stone Age diet used by allergy specialists. If you note a change with your gut after the introduction of one food, then you know that you are intolerant to that food and you should stay away. Do not be too quick to introduce a new food into your diet. It takes about three days to know if the last food was something that was bad for your gut. All that three days to pass before you introduce yet another food so that you do not have confusing results.

When you find that you are left in doubt, put the food to one side and try to introduce it at a later date to see whether it causes reactions.

So what can you eat now after getting rid of all the above foods? Let us have a look at that.

(k) What To Take

The foods you are allowed to eat only apply if you don't have intolerance to them. You can have an intolerance test to know the food you are intolerant to or you can try the above method of introduction to eliminate those that you are intolerant to. Only take what your body is okay with even though they are accepted in the diet. Here are some of the foods:

Meats and eggs

The best choice of meat you should eat is from pastured and grass fed animals from a local farm. These are fish, beef, organ meats, chicken, lamb etc. Meats from factory-farmed animals should be avoided since they contain hormones and antibiotics. For the eggs, you should preferably buy free-range organic eggs since they don't have chemicals and antibiotics coming into contact with them. They are also superior in their nutritional value.

You should never use packaged and commercial meat stock. The meat should be eaten with collagen and fat so you should avoid lean meat. You should also not purchase preserved meats.

It is important to also know that meat and fish should be taken with vegetables because the acidity that comes with digesting meat and alkalinity from vegetables balances each other out. You should mostly eat the organs, bones, skin and marrows since they have collagen, which will help in rebuilding of your digestive lining. As we stated earlier, the lining of the digestive tubes will have been affected by your bad diet and leaky gut is a direct consequence of this. Thus, you need to rebuild that lining as quickly as possible to help you to gain the real benefits from your food.

Most vegetables

Except the starchy ones like sweet potatoes and potatoes, you can take asparagus, beets, celery, garlic, zucchini, rhubarb, watercress, lettuce, carrots, onions, squash etc. Non-starch vegetables are recommended since the more the starch a vegetable has, the more sugar it contains which feed pathogenic bacteria as well as cause surges in your blood sugar levels. All the vegetables should be organic since they contain fewer pesticides and other toxic chemicals. If this means buying them at a farmer's market, it will be more expensive, but it's worth it. If you can consider growing your own for the future, you can avoid this extra expense. The benefits far outweigh the inconvenience of price since by buying a local farm produce stands, you actually do a lot of good for your body, for the environment as well as knowing where your foods come from. The tastes that you will enjoy will be better than the taste of vegetables which have gone through processes or which have been sprayed with hormones during the course of their growth. You will also come into contact with new vegetables that you may not have tried and that will really get the taste buds going.

Fruits, which are low in glycemic

Many people would suggest that you completely stop eating most of the fruits, but this is not always necessary. You can have fruit in moderation, and you should always aim for low glycemic foods.

- Banana.
- Cherries.
- Prunes.
- Grapefruit.
- Apples.
- Plums.
- Mangoes.
- Kiwi Fruit.
- Pears

You will notice that the cross section of fruit that you can eat is good, meaning that you have a variety for cooking and for eating raw. That's good news for juicers too because you have enough contrast of taste to produce super smoothies within the parameters of the diet.

Herbs and Spices

Apart from meats and vegetables, what you also need to add into your dishes is herbs and spices. If you are not allowed to add some basic herbs into your foods, the dishes would not taste the same. It is acknowledged that herbs can also be beneficial to the body and in fact aid digestion. That means that experimentation is going to help you to retain really good flavors. The Natural Society backs these as being beneficial and if you have never used some of the spices and herbs shown below, read up on their uses as they really can enhance the taste of your food.

Here's the list of spices that are a good fit for your condition:
- Basil
- Garlic
- Ginger
- Cinnamon
- Salt (Non-Iodized)
- Chives
- Cilantro

- Sage
- Saffron
- Oregano
- Mint
- Marjoram
- Dill
- Turmeric
- Thyme

Herbal teas

Particularly green tea. Some of the teas that are beneficial to your health are particularly those such as mint tea, which aids digestion. Do read labels and don't just buy because it says it's an herb tea. These are best bought from natural sources such as health food stores, rather than buying cheap brands in the supermarket. One tea that is particularly beneficial and may be bought in dried format from the pharmacy is white nettle. This is a great detox tea and is useful when treating the gut health.

Animal fats and oils

Butter, lard, ghee (clarified butter) and duck fats. The best are natural fats from meats. They are also amazing to cook with because they don't change their chemical structure when they are being heated.

Avocado oil, flax seed oil, olive oil and evening primrose oil are great to dress salads with but they should not be used for cooking because this will destroy their nutrients. If you have never used duck fat, prepare for a feast, because its taste is superb.

Coconut

Coconut milk, coconut oil, coconut cream and coconut butter could work.

Beans and pulses

They should be introduced slowly into the diet since they are hard to digest. You should also ensure that you soak dry beans, peas and lentils for at least 12 hours. After that, drain them and rinse them under running water to eliminate harmful substances e.g. lectins. The only kinds of beans allowed are lima, string, white or haricot beans, lentils and split beans. The rest have too much starch. These are great for thickening otherwise boring broth and with added herbs, you really can make a tasty stew.

Fats

You should favor the consumption of fat over

carbohydrates, as fat will give you a more stable blood sugar and thus prevent low-level inflammation. Fat is also important for your endocrine function, because it's essential in the process of hormone production.

Here is a list of fats that, according to a research study, are not harmful to a patient of Hashimoto's:

- Coconut Oil
- Tallow
- Duck Fat
- Lard
- Olive Oil Or Olives
- Avocado Or Avocado oil.

Nuts and seeds: Ensure you buy nuts in their shells or when they are freshly shelled. They should also be raw and not processed, roasted, coated or salted. And due to the fibrous nature of nuts, you should not have them if you are experiencing diarrhea.

Seeds such as sesame and pumpkin are easier to digest if they are soaked in water for about 12 hours.

Honey: This is the only sweetener allowed in the GAPS diet. It should be unheated, unfiltered and raw. Heating will kill the enzymes in the honey. Honey is an antiseptic and it contains many minerals, vitamins and amino acids.

Salt: You should only use whole or crystal sea salt because table salt lacks all the minerals, and this can make the salt detrimental to your health. Examples of crystal salt you could use are Himalayan crystal, Utah salts and sea salts.

During this time, it is very important to have a personal food journal. Use this journal to write what you are eating and how it affects your body. If you feel gassy, bloated or fatigued, add that meal to your elimination list. This is most likely because your body is sensitive to that food.

The elimination diet is helpful but a strict diet is often necessary. Food intolerance and allergies are unreliable and they can't be reliable in the repair of serious digestive issues. The diet can be followed for around 10-60 days or longer for extensive repair. You could even adopt the diet to feel better and function at your best. This diet is also proved to reverse acute intolerance to substances like gluten and eggs. You should also try to do away with any misconception you have about good food (for example low fat diets). Also, ensure that you find out the truth from marketing claims about food so that you don't end up consuming food that will be harmful to your body in the end.

So, what next after getting rid of foods that are causing you problems and introducing better foods? The next step is replacing.

Step 2: Replace

The next step would be to provide your body with what is needed in order to repair the gut lining. This includes:

Digestive enzymes

You should take a lot of digestive enzymes for breaking down the food you consume. Leaky gut needs crucial enzyme support for healing and rebuilding villi. You should take enzyme supplements just before taking a meal to jumpstart digestion. There are natural enzymes in honey but they may be insufficient for your needs. However, it's worth bearing in mind that mango also contains digestive enzymes. Fenugreek tea can help you with providing enzymes, although there are arguments between experts as to the efficiency of bought pills. Thus, it would be wise to opt for those enzymes which can be derived from what you eat rather than getting on the bandwagon and finding that you are taking unnecessary pills that you later feel you cannot do without. Added to this, drinking sufficient water is useful to aid the digestion.

Omega -3 fatty acids

You should consume more omega-3 fatty acids because the gut uses them for rebuilding healthy cells and to calm inflammation. Some of the recommended omega 3 foods are nuts, avocadoes, cold water fish, seeds and purslane. Try to include cold water fish at least three times a week because these really are rich in Omega 3 fatty acids and are easy to incorporate into your menu for the week.

Whole foods

You should eat plenty of whole foods. Whole foods are full of phytonutrients, minerals enzymes and vitamins that the small intestine requires in order to heal. As your body detoxifies, it will need a lot of fiber in order to get rid of the byproducts and toxins through the large intestine as fast as possible. Foods with a lot of fiber include colorful veggies, seeds, nuts, legumes, etc. As we have already stated, if you do opt for greens such as broccoli, make sure that they are cooked well.

Glutamine

You should supplement with glutamine since it is a free amino acid and it supports digestion and immunity. Glutamine is known to heal the intestinal lining faster and more than any other nutrient. Since you are not permitted to eat certain foods that provide natural glutamine, it is wise to take a supplement daily to make up for the deficit of glutamine in the digestive tract. This is far better than cheating and including banned foods based on the reasoning that they contain glutamine. There are reasons for the elimination of certain foods and as glutamine is perfectly safe in capsule format, this also allows you to see the exact amount taken per day.

Step 3: Introducing Healthy Bacteria

Once your gut has patched up all the leaks, you need to make it stronger by increasing the good gut bacteria. Below are ways of achieving this:

Add a probiotic in your diet

Probiotics are important for rejuvenating and replenishing micro biomes damaged by poor diet or antibiotics. You should choose a probiotic that is enteric coated because they will carry the bacteria through the acidity of the stomach to the alkaline intestines. Probiotics should come from pharmaceutical-grade supplements and real food. The supplements should contain at least 8 billion cells of bacteria per gram. Do speak to your pharmacy staff and specify that you prefer a probiotic with an enteric coating. Although certain yogurts purport to be probiotics do not be lulled into buying them. The pharmacy will be able to give you the correct product needed.

Eat fermented foods

This is to help your Probiotics to stick around.

Fermented foods also ensure you lower inflammation and improved antioxidant status.

In order to have your gut perfectly in order, you also need to stay calm and keep your central nervous system that way. When you are under stress, your body is in flight or fight mode. You can consider meditation or yoga to assist you in keeping calm.

You should also eat as mindfully as possible. Before you eat, try to take in the aroma of your food to help with the production of enzymes to break down the food. You should also pay attention as you eat and don't multi task. Ensure you savor each bite to avoid any chance of indigestion. Mindfulness is not only popular. It's actually better for your gut health because it means that you chew your food properly instead of expecting the digestive tube to do the work for you.

These include pickled ginger, coconut yogurt, sauerkraut, kimchi, cucumbers that are fermented, kombucha etc. You are supposed to make them for yourself or buy the few brands that are fermented genuinely and not made with added vinegar instead. They should also be free from additives or sugar.

Note:

It is important to know that not all people diagnosed with Hashimoto's require treatment. They could just be monitored for any changes in the functioning of the thyroid gland. If you are not experiencing other difficulties due to Hashimoto's and are happily taking Levothyroxine and finding this sufficient, that's fine.

Removing autoimmune triggers like environmental toxins and infectious agents can help reduce the chances of getting the disease. An example of the environmental exposure can be from rocket fuels, radiation exposure or even polychlorinated.

Acupuncture has also been recently proved to regulate the immune responses Th1 and Th2. It helps in managing the thyroid function but you should not avoid treatment because of this. If you keep having your blood tests at regular intervals and it is seen that acupuncture has helped, your doctor may be able to adjust your medications.

Some essential fatty acids are also known to reduce inflammation caused by the disease. The fatty acids can be regulated to reduce inflammation by increasing intake of Omega 3 fats and reducing intake of omega 6 fats.

Administering selenium could also work. It has been found to increase the thyroid function by reducing thyroid antibodies. Seafood, sunflower seeds and Brazil nuts have selenium in them.

Study has also showed that lower level laser therapy has also been found to be effective as it improves the function of the thyroid. If you are going to consider this, consult a specialist.

We will have a look at some simple recipes that you can prepare to get started on getting rid of Hashimoto's by embracing a suitable diet.

Sample Recipes

Here are some recipes prepared from the allowed foods in the GAPS diet. Remember to use the ingredients in the conditions they are permitted to be used in. The recipes are a cross section and you will find many more if you simply look through the pages of Pinterest where people who are on this diet have been sharing their favorite recipes. Remember to batch bake and freeze many of the recipes so that you are ready for your diet and can easily have food available, as that really is half of the battle when changing your diet to help your Hashimoto's disease.

Elimination Diet- Friendly Almond Bread

Makes 1 loaf

Ingredients

4 ½ tablespoons of water
¼ teaspoon of pure sea salt
1 tablespoon of coconut oil
1 ½ tablespoons of ground flax seeds

1 ¼ cups of almond flour
1 teaspoon of baking soda
1 tablespoon of honey

Directions

Preheat the oven to 300 degrees. Put the flax seeds in a bowl, add water and mix well. Leave it until it starts forming a gel. Grease the baking pan at the bottom with the coconut oil. Mix the baking soda, salt and flour together.

Add coconut oil and honey into the same bowl that has the flax seeds in it and mix them together well. Pour all the wet ingredients into the dry ones.

Bake for about 30 – 40 minutes or until the bread is golden brown and when you insert a tooth pick into it, it comes out clean. But make sure you do not burn it! If your oven is one where even temperature is a problem, turn the bread half way through cooking to ensure even cooking.

Almond Flour Zucchini Pancakes

Yields about 6 pancakes

This is a recipe that is worthwhile getting familiar with to make sure that you always have the ingredients in the home. Remember that quick recipes are okay for those times when you have time to cook and among the recipes given, pancakes are a favorite for those days when you really don't want to do a huge amount of cooking.

Ingredients

1 small zucchini, grated
1 cup of almond flour
½ teaspoon of sea salt
3 sprigs of fresh thyme- chopped
1 tablespoon of honey (raw and unheated)
1 small apple, grated
2-3 tablespoons of almond butter (or you can use any butter really)
3 eggs
2 tablespoons of coconut oil

Directions

Combine the zucchini, apples, almond butter, honey and thyme in a bowl. Combine the baking powder, flour and salt in a different bowl. Beat the eggs lightly and then combine all the ingredients. Heat the coconut oil in the pan and fry the pancakes for about 5 minutes on every side but make sure not to burn to them. If you haven't tried almond flour, this will become a clear favorite for your baking needs.

Baked Stuffed Pumpkin

Serves 4-6

Ingredients

2 cups of cooked brown rice
1 ½ cups of cranberries
2 teaspoons of salt
2 stalks of sage (chopped)
1 medium sized pumpkin
1 cup of chopped pecans
1 cup of chicken stock
2 tablespoons flax seed meal- ground flax seeds
2 tablespoons of olive oil

Directions

Preheat your oven to 200 degrees. As it heats, cut the pumpkin at the top and seed it. Rub the outer side of the pumpkin with olive oil. Combine all ingredients in a bowl to make the stuffing. Stuff the pumpkin and cover the top with the pumpkin top. Place it in a tray and set it in your pre heated oven to bake for about an hour or until very soft and serve!

GAPS Ultimate Soup

Serves 6

Ingredients

10 ounces sugar snap peas
10 ounces asparagus
4 cups water
3 tablespoons of brown rice
2 tablespoons of olive oil
½ cup of fresh mint leaves -loosely packed
2-3 tablespoons fresh lemon juice, more to taste

Freshly ground black pepper- to taste
10 ounces of fennel bulbs
1 bunch of green onions (the white and green parts)
1 ½ teaspoons of sea salt
2 large leeks
½ cup of fresh dill, loosely packed
3 cups of light vegetable broth/ chicken broth
Grated lemon peel from one lemon
Fruity green olive oil for garnish

Directions

Wash the vegetables and then string then coarsely chop all the snap peas, and chop the fennel bulbs and slice the green onions and asparagus. Add all the vegetables, rice, water and a teaspoon of salt to a large pot and simmer for about 30 minutes. As it simmers, chop the green onions. Sauté the onions in olive oil with salt over medium oil for about 20 minutes. Add the broth, mint, dill and cooked onions to the vegetables. After the soup has simmered for a few minutes set it to cool. Puree the ready soup in a blender until smooth. Return it to the pot then add sea salt, lemon juice and pepper to taste.

Granola Snack

This is also a useful snack to have in stock so try to bulk bake so that you have plenty. At least that way, you can have a snack between meals without cheating on your diet.

Serves 2

Ingredients

½ cup of almonds, sliced
½ cup of pumpkin seeds
¼ cup of coconut oil
2 teaspoons of cinnamon
½ cup of dried apricots- chopped
1 cup of pecans, chopped
1 cup of coconut, shredded
¼ cup of honey
½ teaspoon of nutmeg

Directions

Preheat your oven to 350 degrees. Grease the bottom of the baking sheet with coconut oil. Mix well all ingredients except the dried fruit. Spread the ingredients evenly on the greased baking sheet. Bake for about 15 minutes as you stir it occasionally. Remove and stir in the dried apricots.

Goji Grapefruit Parsley Smoothie

First of all, just to let you know which nutrients you are going to have in your smoothie, I will make you a list and then will give you a little detail about them. These are all relevant when it comes to treating Hashimoto's disease or other immune diseases and will help you make sure that you get sufficient of the different vitamins and minerals that your body need.

- Selenium
- Vitamin C
- Iron
- Zinc
- Calcium
- Potassium
- Riboflavin.

Selenium is one of the key minerals that most of the patients of Hashimoto's are deficient in, therefore, when you add 50 grams of dried wolfberries containing 25 micrograms (50% DRI), you will get a good amount of selenium in it. Your body needs 55 mcg of selenium per day. Bananas, raisins and dried dates also contain selenium meaning that you can use a variety of fruit in your smoothies. Berries are the best source which is why this was mentioned first although you can expect to get 1.0 mcg from a cup full of raisins, 1.5 from a cup of sliced banana and as high as 4.4 from dates. However, small quantities of dates are preferred in a smoothie because of the sugar content.

Riboflavin, which is also a source of vitamin B2, is again in wolfberries.

Vitamin C will provide 16% and 82% DRI.

Wolfberries have 4.5 mg **iron** per 50 grams, thus providing 50% DRI.

Ingredients

1 cup of filtered water
Handful of almonds
Handful of pecans
Handful of walnuts
1 tbsp. of milk thistle
1.5 tbsp. of ground flax seed (flax seed meal)
Handful of hemp seeds

Handful of fresh parsley
½ grapefruit
Handful of dry goji berries that must be soaked

Directions

First of all, you need to soak the goji berries for two hours or at least two hours or overnight. Then you need to blend all the ingredients with the help of your blender. It depends on you if you want it to be blended completely, or if you would prefer some chunks in it. It would hardly take seven minutes for it preparation. Only the berries would take some hours for them to get perfectly soaked. Then serve yourself the delicious smoothie in a fine glass, and tell yourself it is for your own good. Enjoy!

What is special about A Goji grapefruit parsley smoothie?

You can have it in your breakfast, in your lunch, or in your dinner. This is going to be very healthy and nutritious for you, as it contains most of the minerals that your body requires in Hashimoto's. As there are some nuts in this shake, you'll need to try to see if your body will tolerate them. Remember, you can vary the smoothie a little by adding the recommended fruits listed above under the heading of selenium.

Homemade Ginger Ale

Another one of our most favorite recipe is Ginger Ale. The fact that it is delicious as well as nutritious raises its value to a great degree. Also, it will only take very little of your time to prepare it. And it is not at all difficult to prepare. You can find the ingredients easily in your nearby supermarket. Having a stock of this will help as well because it's a good alternative to unhealthy caffeine based drinks such as coffee.

Ingredients

First, you need to get enough filtered water to fill the jar.
Two large pinches of unrefined sea salt
take 2 tbsp. raw whey
take 1/4th cup of lime juice
take 3-6 tbsp. raw honey
and lastly, take ½ cup of ginger root.

Directions

The method to make it is fairly simple. You need to take care of only some things before you make it. For example, the fresh ginger root should be peeled and grated. Then you have to make sure that the root is moist and aromatic. It should not be dried out. The raw honey that you are going to add in it should be very soft and not hot at all. The fresh limejuice made from about 1-4 limes should be made, but keep in check the juiciness of the lime. Other than that, you need to bring the limes to room temperature before juicing for best results. Raw whey is perfect the way it is; it does not require anything to be done to it before its usage. And, in fact, that is pretty much it!

Now you need to know about the procedure to make it. It is as simple as the ingredients were. All you need to do is to combine all the ingredients in a glass jar that measures one-quarter. Covering it with the screw lid, you need to shake it up gently enough so that the honey gets dissolved. Then leave it at room temperature for almost a day i.e., 24 hours. Then you have to strain it into two 25.3 oz. Pellegrino bottles with screw-on lids. Lastly, top it off both with Pellegrino, and then simply store it in the refrigerator until it is cooled. You are ready to enjoy your homemade ginger ale.

Blackberry Power Smoothie

Have you ever tried a blackberry smoothie before? Are you a big fan? Or have you never tried it? In either case, you have a chance once again to enjoy the unique flavor of a blackberry power smoothie, which could be made in only one minute. It has the high protein amount, high fat, and high fiber. Another plus is that it had low sugar, which is highly prohibited for a Hashimoto's patient. It will make you feel satisfied and nourished just the second you take the last sip of it.

Ingredients

1 tbsp. raw honey (however, it is optional)
1 tbsp. of pumpkin seed (It really depends on you if you want it or not)
1 tbsp. of coconut oil or coconut ghee
1 cup of warm water (make sure it is warm)
half tsp Camu Camu powder
1 tbsp. of milk whistle
one and a half tbsps. of ground flax seed (flax seed meal)
And lastly, a handful of organic blueberries

Method

Take all these ingredients, and blend them all together in your blender. Next, you have to see if you like chunks in it or not. If you do not like chunks, then you would have to blend it as long as it looks completely smooth to the naked eye. If it is difficult to detect, you can stir the solution with the help of a spoon and detect if there are any chunks left or not. The last step is to turn off the blender, pour it in a beautiful glass, grab some snacks, and go outside on your lawn and sip it while you're basking in the sun (if you have not forgotten how good sunlight is for you in giving you vitamins). It is the easiest recipe of a smoothie among all the recipes that we have introduced to you or will later in this chapter. It is as easy to make as it is to consume. You can also serve it to your guests while you are enjoying it.

Kabocha Squash and Celery Root Soup

Enough with the drinks. Now I think we should try some edibles too, although technically, soup is not to be eaten or chewed. But it can be placed in the mixed category, since it sometimes has corn and chicken in it.

Ingredients

3 tbsp. unsalted butter
hot paprika or chili could be used as its
substitute
for garnishing, you can use pumpkin seeds
4 cups of chicken stock
juice of 1 lemon and the skin zest
1 sprig of rosemary which should be finely
chopped
1 sprig of sage which should be finely chopped
2 leeks which should be fine chopped
1 and a half teaspoon of sea salt
2 tbsp. of coconut oil
2 tbsp. of beef tallow or duck fat
1 large celery root which must be peeled and
finely chopped to 1-inch cubes
1 kabocha squash (2 and a half lb. or1 + kg). It
should be peeled and cubed if they are to be cooked,
or else they should be cut in halves in case they are
to be roasted.

Method

Here are 9 simple steps to make this delicious
Kabocha Squash and Celery Root Soup

As discussed above in the ingredients, if you are

aiming to roast the squash and the celery for one hour, then roast it until it gets really soft or if you are going to peel the skin off, then it is better for you to cook it right away in the pot. Both the methods bear their own advantages. Roasting will make it easy to scoop out the flesh, but we warn you that this method will take a long time to be prepared. However, cooking will only ask of you to peel the skin off which you might not like to do or you might not.

Anyhow, if you are roasting, then you need to preheat the oven up to 400 F and place the squash halves face down on the parchment paper. And then you can add celery root cubes on it. Then roast the veggies for 45 to 65 minutes straight, and keep checking when it gets soft with the help of a fork.

Then you have to keep a check on the coconut oil when you melt it in a pan, and the leeks and sauté onions that you add with it. Cook them until they get really soft and brown, but do not burn them away.

Now this is the time when you add herbs, salt, roasted squash, celery roots, and chicken stock in it. However, if you are not roasting them, then just add them raw.

Simmer for 1 hour if raw, or 20 minutes if it is roasted.

Add butter, chili, zest, and lemon juice.

When it is cooled, blending them in a food processor or the blender till it gets very smooth.

Here is the best part: garnishing! You can use pumpkin seeds to garnish the freshly prepared soup. After all you have done, what is there left to do? Eating the yummy soup! Seize it!

Now you can enjoy your homemade Kabocha Squash and Celery Root Soup. The best part is, it is very easy and quick to make. Its preparation time is just twenty-five minutes, and the cooking time is only one hour if it is cooked, and one and a half hour if you are planning to roast it, and also, it can serve 7-8 people at a time!

Baked Stuffed Pumpkin

Here is one last recipe that you will thoroughly enjoy. It is as simple as the other recipes were. And yes, this one is absolutely eatable, not drinkable. You can serve it to your guests and to you yourself since it is not specifically for a Hashimoto's patient. Anyone can enjoy it as much as you can. Here is a quick recipe:

Ingredients

2 tbsp. olive oil
2 stalks of sage that must be chopped.
2 tbsp. of flaxseed meal which must be grounded
2 teaspoon of salt
one and a half cup of cranberries
1 cup chicken stock
1 cup of pecans which should also be chopped
2 cups of rice which should be cooked
And lastly, one medium sized pumpkin in which you are going to fill everything in.

Method

Here are few steps to make this recipe

First of all, make sure that you preheat the oven for maximum 400F or 200C.

Then grab that middle-sized pumpkin, cut the top of it off with a sharp knife, and then scoop out all the seeds in it. Olive oil should be applied on its outer surface.

Now take a bowl and add all the ingredients given above. Mix them up.

Now that you have stuffed the pumpkin with every ingredient, cover the top of it with the pumpkin top.

Place that stuffed pumpkin on a tray and bake it in 400F oven for an hour or until it gets really soft. Keep checking it by poking it with the help of a fork.

Just the second your oven rings the bell, open it up and take out the delicious, perfectly cooked pumpkin, and then serve it on a dish. You can serve it both ways, as a side dish or a main dish. It would only take 25 minutes for its preparation and one hour to be cooked in a soft texture. You can serve to up to 6 to 8 people. Not only would you enjoy it, but also the people accompanying you at that dining table.

All the recipes given above sound very delicious. But once you try them, you would know the fact that not only they are delicious but also, highly nutritious. All you need to keep in your notice is that no prohibited food items get accidentally added in your recipes, because if that happens, then all the effect it has to produce in your body might unintentionally be reversed.

Although this diet is very restrictive, it really is worthwhile watching the video from its founder because it makes a lot of sense and can actually relieve a lot of discomfort and make your bodywork better long term. It's strict for a purpose. If you care more for your health and wellbeing than you care about the initial inconvenience, then this is the diet that will help your Hashimoto's long term and is a good investment because of how healthy you will feel when not subjecting your body to things that it really wasn't intended to digest long term. Plus the fact that food intolerances play a huge part in how you feel anyway – this diet makes sense for those who know that their digestive system is causing a lot of problems.

Why the Paleo Diet Can be a Viable Alternative

You may be wondering why we included details on two diets. There is a very good reason for this. In today's world, people are so accustomed to eating prepared foods that it's hard to follow a more restrictive diet long term without actually cheating even if this is unintentional. The GAPS diet is restrictive, but it's restrictive for very good reason. The doctor who explains the diet can do a much better job of this than I can in explaining why this diet has been formulated and when you hear about the success that it has had with all kinds of illnesses, then it's a very serious step, but you may not be ready for that step. The Paleo diet, on the other hand, can be followed at times when you know your gut really is suffering due to your Hashimoto's and can help you to get it back to working condition so that you don't suffer leaky gut more than you have to.

There are also other reasons why the Paleo diet is so successful. In a way, it educates people about what they are subjecting their bodies to. If you follow the Paleo diet and become familiar with how it works for your body, you may even find yourself incorporating elements from it into your normal diet to help avoid the kind of problems that modern foods are causing to your gut.

The diet is explained in the next chapter, but if you are thinking of following it, make sure that you have lots of stock in the house and that those who are not following the diet are aware that they won't be doing you any favors if they insist on offering you tempting foods that are not on that diet sheet. The way to do this is to make them aware that you are doing this for health purposes and you will gain their support. Often, with weight loss diets, people tempt you to actually justify their own eating habits. If you have told people that you have a lot of health problems, then usually they are more encouraging and will help you along the way.

I would suggest that you keep your diet food separate from the food that is to be used for others, so that you have clear cut ideas about what you can and cannot include. Try to avoid jumping into the diet too quickly because if you do, you may find that you don't stick to it for the set amount of time that you have planned. The reason for this is the lack of preparation. When faced with a choice of making something or grabbing something from a ready-made packet, let's face it, the packets seem very tempting. Thus, preparation and slow introduction to the diet is probably the best way to incorporate Paleo at the beginning. When you think of how long it took you to learn your current eating habits, you can't expect to be able to change those overnight. However, what you can do is start your preparations and incorporate a few Paleo items into your diet gradually, so you become accustomed to the different choices and actually allow your taste buds to get used to the different recipes. There is a particular cookie recipe that my family enjoys more than bought cookies and thus they now expect this as part of their family mealtime treats. That's a good thing because it means that you are taking in one less problematic food and that's always an improvement.

You need to set a time for your diet. Thus, a thirty day diet wouldn't be unreasonable to think about and have things planned in advance. That month may be all it takes to help mend your digestive tube so that it no longer bloats and you feel much better because the lining has been able to replenish itself which is what modern foods don't allow it to do. Paleo diet foods need to be recognized easily before you start your 30 days, so familiarize yourself with the foods and work out menus for the whole 30 days.

One thing that is rather neat on the Paleo diet is that you can fast from time to time and you may even feel energized from it. If you try intermittent fasting, that means you have less preparation to do and can help your body to detox by drinking nettle tea during the fasting period. That's a great eliminator and will help you to feel much better. Hashimoto's tends to make you feel very sluggish, bloated up and lethargic about life and by doing this, you awaken your taste buds and also give your body the rest it deserves meaning that your gut gets a great clean out between foods.

If you phase out bad foods one at a time, it makes the transition to Paleo a lot easier to handle and then at the beginning of the 30 days, plunge into the diet with a new enthusiasm, using only Paleo approved foods. During the phasing out period, how about enthusing yourself by cleaning out all your kitchen cupboards of junk or foods that are disallowed? This helps the preparation and you can remind yourself why you need to do this and reinforce it by ditching those foods which really are making your health worse.

The first thing to remember with the Paleo diet is that you need to detox your gut at the very beginning to help the Paleo foods to do their thing. Thus, having nettle tea ready by the bottle full is a good idea. If you boil water and put in the prepared nettles from the health food shop, you can actually do a quantity at a time and bottle it so that you always have it on hand to drink and detox in the early stages of the Paleo diet. The foods that you have been eating may have created small pockets in your digestive tract and the detox will help to sort this out as well as preparing you for your new diet.

Spend a good deal of time researching and getting information on foods and recipes that you feel will help you in your Paleo diet. There are loads online and Pinterest has a lot that can give ideas of meals when your ideas run out. It's best to do the research before you start because otherwise you can't really make the best meal plan and without that meal plan, you are likely to be tempted into going back to old ways. The recipes included with this book are just the beginning. There are thousands of alternatives that you can have and the more ideas you glean, the better your chances of success.

Remember that the better you learn this diet, the

better you are equipped for future times when you feel that your body is getting sluggish again. You will be ready to change what you eat because you will have already experienced the benefits and believe me, they are many. I like the fact that the Paleo diet actually educates you about the things that you are eating now that may actually be harming you, even though they may be labeled in such a way as to tempt you into buying them – thinking that you are buying healthy alternatives when in fact, you are buying into the hype.

Changing your mind set on diets

You need to change your mind set before you start the initial thirty days. You need to stop thinking of this in the traditional way that people view diets. Instead, think of it as your Hashimoto cure. You are doing this for your health. You are not doing this with expectations of weight loss. Weight loss will probably happen anyway because you will be cutting out a lot of the junk that you currently eat, but that shouldn't be the main purpose of the diet. You are doing this because you really don't want to go on suffering. The improvements that you see over the course of eating the right foods should be sufficient incentive to stick to it, but thinking of it as a cure rather than a diet is the healthy mind set to get yourself into.

If you do cheat, don't beat yourself up about it, but don't do it too regularly. Simply get back onto the Paleo diet and keep it going because your gut really will thank you for it. Paleo is used for all kinds of different reasons, but Hashimoto's really will improve when you use the diet because you are in effect fixing your metabolism and that means a great deal when it comes to energy and zest for life.

Even though you may have decided only to do the Paleo thing for thirty days, that may be sufficient to make you feel better and whenever you have a setback, your mind will already know that the Paleo diet can come to the rescue if you keep notes. I kept notes on how I felt before the Paleo diet and then kept scrupulous notes on how I felt and what I found that this did was actually change my attitude and that's where you need to be to make it work.

Have you ever heard of the placebo effect? You probably have. It's where if your mind believes that something will work, it will. Doctors use it all of the time and whether a diet works for you really does depend upon your belief in it to a certain extent. Stop looking at it as deprivation because it may just lengthen your life and that's hardly a bad thing. Start looking at it as self-improvement and controlling the way that you feel without relying too heavily on medications.

You need most of all to believe in your own strength of character because when push comes to shove, that's what any diet is all about. The thing is that when it relates to your health and wellbeing, you need to remind yourself of what you stand to gain and thoroughly believe in it. I remember

Hashimoto's making me very constipated and bloated and it only took three days for a Paleo diet to actually fix that. Taking medications for constipation on a regular basis is extremely unhealthy. In fact, on most boxes of meds for constipation, there is a warning that you should adjust your diet or seek medical help if you find that you need to take constipation medications more regularly than once in a while. You may even be sabotaging your health if this is the way that you run your life, thinking that you can overcome gut problems in this way. Paleo puts a stop to that and when you find yourself becoming regular, the bloating goes down and you feel much more energetic.

Make Paleo foods cheaper

A lot of people say that Paleo foods are more expensive and they can be. You are expected to buy fresh foods and meats and these cost money. However, if you have plenty of room in the freezer, you can take advantage of sales of fresh farm meat. Often, you can pick up bulk food a lot cheaper than going out shopping on a regular basis. Thus this helps you considerably. If you know that you will use Paleo foods in the future, then it may be worthwhile investing in a bit of hard work to get your garden going so that you can be surer of the freshness of your foods. If you have enough land, try some free range eggs. Eggs are a great source of protein and if you have chickens, you will know that the chickens were fed on good quality feed.

When I was researching the diet for my Hashimoto's I remember seeing a website that gave information that I found amusing but which turned out to be very true indeed. If you have seen the product advertised on TV, then you can be pretty sure it's not Paleo!

Snacks help you to keep on track

I tended to plan a couple of meals a day and in between time was content with snacks of the Paleo ilk. Make sure that you get these ready at the weekend or on an evening when you have plenty of time. That way, if the hunger pangs kick in, at least you have the option of Paleo snacks. Boiled eggs in the fridge mean that you have an instant breakfast. Invest in a poacher since cooking eggs in this manner means delicious breakfasts or the potential to use these for a light evening meal.

Making Paleo Fun

I can hear you now complaining at that heading. How can you make a diet fun? Well, the fact is that you can. I am sure that the Stone Age people who ate Paleo didn't really think in the same way as we do because they didn't have alternatives. However, you do. Use these to their best advantage to make the cure fun. I say cure because we need to get away from thinking of this as some kind of diet because people always associate negativity with diets. Think of the improvements it will make for you and try some fun ideas to make it seem more enjoyable.

You can have ketchup – make your own and be satisfied that it's a modern introduction but one that will really give your food taste.

Eating bacon is very enjoyable and on the Paleo diet, you can eat as much as you like!

Challenge yourself – There are loads of Paleo equivalents for food that you are accustomed to eating. Challenge the family to find them so that you can give them a try and then your diet will seem very similar to what you are accustomed to eating. All you are doing is substituting foods.

Grow fresh herbs in pots with your kids. Let them see the benefit of growing them and tasting what they have helped you to grow. They really will get more enthusiastic about it if they have taken part in the preparation.

Get the kids to help with preparing the food. You can even talk about the Stone Age and explain to the kids the reasons why Stone Age food wasn't such a bad idea. If you consider your cure period as a time to educate the kids, you may actually persuade them to eat healthier choices. Look at labels together and make notes of the enemies. Colorants and E numbers in any kind of quantity can make people very sick. Thus make this a fun time with the kids and let them learn from an early age what it good for you and what is not.

Have plenty of nuts of the healthy varieties available for snacks. Deprivation is not what it's about. It's about improving your Hashimoto's, but there's no reason why kids can't learn good food preparation ideas from you because they may actually find the Paleo diet will be useful to them in the future.

The preparation that you put into the diet is vital to success. Don't think that you can suddenly change over to another kind of diet without this preparation because it's not as easy as you think and buying food from the supermarket may be tempting if you don't prepare. Thus, if you want to give the most benefit to your body, then it's essential to give the diet the best chance possible of lasting by researching, collecting recipes, understanding the food groups that you are permitted and making the most of creating your weekly menu, which also enables you to get all the supplies in that you are likely to need. If you doubt your discipline, Paleo is going to be an easier option to GAPS. However, if you have good discipline, GAPS is the long term answer to your problems with Hashimoto's disease.

What people are saying about the Paleo diet

The Paleo diet has been around for long enough to have great feedback from people who have used it. I think that this section may help you to make up your mind if you have not already done so. One patient had this to say about the Paleo diet.

"I was worried about the change, but I was more worried about the effect that Hashimoto's disease was having on my body. It took a lot of work but at the end of 30 days, I wondered if I should stick to the Paleo diet permanently! The reason for this was the fact that for the first time in years, a lot of the problems I had which were associated with Hashimoto's actually disappeared and I felt very young and energetic again – for the first time in ages."

If you need the validation of seeing what other people think of the Paleo diet, you only have to do Google searches to find out what people are saying and most of it is positive. There are the people who have difficulty in finding enough variety, but that's only because they are accustomed to the availability of pre-prepared food and are unwilling to go back to basics. The problem is that you can't do it by halves. You need to make up your mind to give it a chance, even if it is inconvenient and make it as convenient as you can for your lifestyle, using your spare time to produce foods ready for the days when you are too busy.

Another lady who tried this said: "My kids got

particularly interested in Paleo because of its history. We were able to combine lessons with cooking and this greatly helped to produce loads of snacks ready for the week that were healthy choices."

Did any of them cheat? Yes, of course they did, but they didn't get hung up about it and as soon as they admitted that they had cheated, they went back onto the diet and tried again and then succeeded. Don't make it punishment. Make it a challenge and if you don't meet the challenge first time, try again.

"I thought that I had fibromyalgia. I thought it would never be cured. However, when I took to the Paleo diet, the pain was much less and I was a lot more mobile."

This lady hadn't been accustomed to incorporating sufficient water into her diet and this helped considerably. With the introduction of water and particularly detox drinks made from nettles, she found that her muscles didn't feel so tired and that she was able to take up sports with her friends with little difficulty. Her metabolism seemed to change and that gave her the energy that she needed to give her the extra push toward giving herself sufficient exercise. That would have been impossible under normal circumstances.

There's a lot of goodness to be gleaned from either the GAPS or the Paleo diet but you need to decide that this is a choice, rather than a punishment because if you start to feel negative about the foods that you eat, you begin to feel deprived. Instead of feeling deprived, consider yourself privileged to be able to take such a courageous step in a world where people are so busy taking the easy way out.

"I cheated," one woman admitted. "I cheated because I could, but the only person I cheated long term was myself. Having gotten over that, I learned that my body really would thank me for the fact that I persevered."

These are testimonies from people with Hashimoto's disease who were able to regain such a lot of their vitality by changing that they were able to forget for a while that they had the disease. Some have chosen to use the GAPS diet on a permanent basis while others have decided to opt for an occasional 30 day Paleo diet when the body seemed to be sluggish and in need of a little help. Using it either way will help, so you need to make the choice yourself depending upon your own lifestyle. It's a personal choice and one that only you can make.

The Paleo Plan – An Introduction

It is a well-established fact that Hashimoto's Thyroiditis is one of many autoimmune diseases that get triggered by an unbalanced lifestyle and an overactive immune system. General concerns of autoimmune patients include:

- Knowing what to eat and what not to eat,
- Repairing a leaky gut,
- Balancing out the immune system,
- Cooling down inflammation,
- Reducing symptoms of diseases like stress, insomnia, etc.

Research has been showing for quite some time now that there are certain foods and bacteria that generate inflammation in the body, especially in the form of intestinal permeability which leads to an autoimmune response that causes the intensity to rise up a notch. Anyone who suffers from any kind of autoimmune disease, including Hashimoto's thyroiditis needs to eliminate all types of foods causing inflammation, heal the intestinal lining and bring back immunity to normal levels. Believe me, you will know when they are out of synch. You will suffer bloating and a very uncomfortable feeling and will not be able to pass stools as quickly as you should. Your gut needs relief from this because keeping food inside you for too long isn't healthy.

Did you know that 80% of your immune system is in your gut? This is exactly why digestive health must be given utmost importance and is therefore the key to a well-managed body. The Paleo Diet Plan that I'm about to share with you has been built to fix your leaky gut by eliminating foods and bacteria that trigger autoimmune reaction in the body. The Plan will rapidly reduce the amount of inflammation the body goes through and heal your body via dietary interventions. In order to calm your immune system down, you'll need to eliminate some food types as well, which comprehensively include grains, nuts, legumes, seeds, alcohol and dairy.

You may need to carry out the plan for 30 days or for as long as the problem persists. Furthermore you will need to realize that your body may contain an overgrowth of yeast, bacteria or other microorganisms, which may be causing an inflammatory response.

In a nutshell, the goal of the diet is to increase anti-inflammatory foods that promote healing while at the same time eliminate the foods that irritate the gut and act as food supplies for bacteria dwelling in the body. By doing so, you will be able to get a control over your body and take care of the Hashimoto's thyroiditis condition that you suffer from. Not only that, you may find that you enjoy the diet and that you want to incorporate it into your lifestyle for longer when you see the benefits that it has.

What Triggers An Autoimmune Response?

You must know that genes and external factors aren't the only thing that drives your body crazy. It has been found that the only reason your body acts like this is due to a solid breach in the intestinal barrier by microorganisms. Leaky gut has been found as the most common cause of this reach and is therefore the 3rd factor that causes diseases like Hashimoto's Thyroiditis.

What is Leaky Gut?

We have already explained this, but need to reinforce what was said, so that you retain this important information. Increased permeability in the intestines is known as leaky gut, which means that opening of the mucosal lining widen resulting in the undigested food bits, bacteria and yeasts to interact with the immune system. Considering the influence a leaky gut has on your immune system, you should always keep the following questions in mind when reading this part of the book:

What triggers leaky gut?

Is it possible to identify and block these irritants?

Can I hack my genes to shut down the response?

What are the symptoms of Leaky gut? These days it is extremely easy to find out whether you suffer from the disease or not, due to the obvious signs of the disease. These include:

- Bloating,
- Poor digestion,
- Multiple foods,
- Chemical insensitivities,
- Inflammation,
- Gut pain,
- Headaches,
- Depression,
- Fatigue and allergies

Moreover, intestinal permeability has been found to link with over a dozen diseases which include autoimmune hepatitis, Celiac disease, Depression, Type 1 diabetes, asthma, Hashimoto's Thyroiditis and many more. The most common triggers of the condition that you'll encounter will include gluten, saponins, alcohol, contraceptives, aspirin, ibuprofen, antibiotics and stress. You need to remember as well that stress can be caused by many different things and that these may be contributing to your condition since you tend to clam up when stress hits and your digestion will be the first thing to be hit by it. People who are depressed can sometimes binge eat and then wonder why the digestive system isn't coping very well. They may also not pay attention to the foods that they are eating and consequently eat all the wrong things.

In addition to these triggers, SIBO and Dysbiosis are also being linked to autoimmune conditions. Dysbiosis is the overgrowth of bacteria, yeast and other parasites in the digestive tract whereas SIBO or small intestinal bacterial overgrowth leads to bloating, diarrhea, constipation and nausea. The toxins involved in SIBO lead to impaired absorption, food intolerances, nutrient deficiencies and antibody responses, all of which contribute to Hashimoto's Thyroiditis.

What is Paleo?

If you're a diet enthusiast then Paleo won't be a stranger to you; if not then let me tell you. The Paleo diet is basically the name given to a lifestyle that was followed by our ancestors long before the advent of modern living techniques like farming, cultivation, etc. They had to rely on themselves and were at the mercy of nature, therefore had to gather food using their bare hands. Moreover, there was no storage mechanism so whatever they ate was fresh and unpolluted. Of course you can't go on hunting trips and follow the Paleo protocol but what you can do is eliminate all foods that weren't available back then. These foods are given in the next chapter and as you read it, you will find out that these are the exact types that cause or worsen the autoimmune condition in the body. Thus, following the diet would automatically bring much needed calmness to the body.

The Plan?

For 30 days or as long as you want to, you will be following a nutrient rich, plant based model that will eliminate the growth of bacteria and other microorganisms while at the same time promote healthy gut conditions. Your blood sugar will stabilize and adrenals will strengthen as your body gets a lot of amino acids and minerals from the proteins and vegetables you consume. Probiotics and cultured foods included in the diet will help bring down intestinal inflammation and promote a better lifestyle in general.

Food Sensitivities

(I) Immunogenic or Allergenic?

There are two types of reactions that your immune system can go through after consuming a particular food. Immunogenic reactions are those that activate some parts of the body's immune system but do not cause an anaphylactic or allergic response; this means that body does not suffer from severe inflammation, making you more sensitive than allergic. There are a number of foods that can be held responsible for such a response that include dairy, gluten, soy, corn and some vegetables. But along with leaky gut, this kind of reaction can soon go undetected and build up to become something really harmful for the body; it can confuse the immune system into thinking that the thyroid tissue is foreign which unleashes an attack on the vital body part.

(m) Cross Reactive Proteins

If you suffer from a sure shot condition of gluten intolerance, then proceed with caution while reintroducing proteins in your diet as some of them may contain chemicals that execute an inflammatory reaction. These cautious proteins are those that are obtained from dairy, oats, yeast, coffee, millet, corn, rice and potato.

(n) Support your Immune System

Basically, what does an autoimmune disease medicine do? It's simple; it works to restore balance to the body's immune system by equalizing the body's hormones. The inflammation loving part of the immune system, known as TH-1, is quick to respond whenever the body is intruded upon, while the anti-inflammatory marker in the body called TH-2, produces antibodies to kill of the invader. In the case of a healthy individual, these two systems work in conjunction and parallel to each other, however, in case of a sick person, these systems go out of order.

Studies are increasingly showing that a new player in the immune system, codenamed TH-17 is making headlines due to its role in protecting the body against these types of diseases. TH-17 is known to activate Nuclear Factor Kappa Beta, which breaks the vicious cycle of inflammation in the body and acts as a permanent solution for the problem.

Coming back to Nuclear Factor Kappa Beta, it is a vital factor when it comes to treating inflammation. Digging a little deeper reveals the real importance of the hormone. SIBO, leaky gut, Dysbiosis and stress are all contributors that trigger NFKB. However, NFKB can be altered with botanicals like curcumin that aid in reducing the effects of inflammation and toning it down a notch.

Curcumin also supports the regulatory T cells, which are responsible for the T hormones stated earlier. When the activity of these cells is regulated, the immune system is kept in check and any unexpected response can be dealt with. This means that a person who suffers from autoimmune diseases like Hashimoto's Thyroiditis can effectively get rid of his/her problem by consuming the right types of foods that pack the right type of nutrients.

This, put in a "nutshell" so to speak, if you follow the Paleo diet, you give your body a chance to recover and to regain its strength and ability to up the metabolism, to feel more energetic, to be able to overcome depression and to also feel much better than you have for a long time. Hashimoto's disease patients have this general feeling of not being well, and when the possibility of feeling good is re-introduced into their lives, it's new hope for people who have perhaps given up hope of ever feeling normal again. You can't get goodness such as that in pill format, but you can get it from changing your eating habits and it's certainly worth doing. With the body complaining about modern foods and showing discomfort from the supply of food that you are giving the gut, now is the best time to do something positive and change the pattern, so that Hashimoto's disease does not rule how you feel. You do.

Next, you will find out the exact food groups

and examples of each that can lead to a healthy Paleo Autoimmune plan.

What to Eat on Paleo?

I'm not going to keep you waiting any longer and jump into the specifics. Here's a list of Do's and Don'ts that you must keep in mind when picking out items at the supermarket or cooking food.

First, the Do's:

- Consume proteins that are pastured, organic and grass fed.
- Eat wild fish not processed ones.
- Carbohydrates obtained from fresh fruits & vegetables would be ideal.
- Consume fruits that have low glycemic content and are low on starch.
- Fermented foods like coconut kefir, sauerkraut and yogurt are allowed.
- Fiber obtained from fruits and vegetables.
- Make colorful vegetables a routine part of your diet.
- Drink at least 8 glasses of water either in raw form or in the form of some broth.
- Exercise for 30 minutes every day, thus mimicking the primitive behavior of our ancestors who had to run, jump and fight for their food.
- Try to meditate at least 5 minutes a day,

- Make green smoothies a part of your diet,
- Sleep at least 7 hours.

Now the don'ts:

- No dairy,
- No grains,
- No wine or alcohol,
- No processed foods,
- No genetically modified food,
- Smoked or salted foods are strictly prohibited,
- Cereals, grains, legumes that include peanuts, lentils, peas, beans and soybeans are
- prohibited.
- Fruit juices containing additives are not allowed.
- Avoid skipping meals.

Allowed Foods

Meats

Poultry	Turkey
Chicken breast	Steak
Ground beef	Grass fed beef
Chicken thigh	Chicken leg
Chicken wings	Lamb rack
Shrimp	Bacon
Pork	Lobster
Clams	Salmon
Venison steaks	Buffalo
Rabbit	Goat
Eggs from ducks, chicken or goose	

You can see from this that you still have a very wide choice and that means you should be able to make yourself menus for a couple of weeks which are varied and interesting. If there are meats in this list that you have never tried, try them! I had never tasted Buffalo, but found it was not dissimilar to beef – but perhaps a little tougher. However, lobster is a real treat and salmon gives you a whole load of possibilities.

Vegetables

Asparagus	Avocado
Artichoke hearts	Brussels sprouts
Carrots	Spinach
Celery	Broccoli
Zucchini	Cabbage
Peppers	Cauliflower
Eggplant	Parsley
Green onions	Butternut squash
Acorn squash	Yam
Sweet Potato	Beets

The vegetable choices here are very useful ones because using these with your meals instead of the standard potato with every meal, you actually learn to enjoy so many different vegetables and may find you continue with them long after the diet is finished.

Fats

- Coconut oil
- Olive oil
- Macadamia oil
- Avocado oil
- Grass fed butter

Don't be afraid of experimentation. You may never have used these oils before but they are delicious and very easy to use. Not only that – they are healthy.

Nuts

- Almonds
- Cashews
- Hazelmuts
- Pecans
- Pine nuts
- Pumpkin seeds
- Sunflower seeds
- Macadamia nut
- Walnuts

Walnuts will become a strong favorite for all kinds of dishes because they are so versatile and sunflower seeds are useful as a snack. Pecans are absolutely delicious. Get to try each of them and find your favorites but remember that unsalted varieties of nuts are the ones that you need to stick to.

Fruits

- Apple
- Avocado
- Blackberries
- Papaya
- Peaches plums
- Mango
- Lychee
- Blueberries
- Grapes
- Lemon
- Strawberries
- Watermelon
- Pineapple guava
- Lime
- Raspberries
- Cantaloupe
- Tangerine
- Oranges
- Bananas

That's a wonderful range of fruits and berries are particularly useful. Since these cover all seasons, it doesn't matter what time of year you start your diet. However, you can freeze in season fruit and use them in your cooking, such as wild blackberries as these are delicious mixed with blanched apples.

Prohibited Foods

Dairy

- Butter
- Cheese
- Non-fat deiry creamer
- Skimme mild
- Whole milk
- Cream cheese
- Dairy spreads
- Lowdered mild
- Yogurt
- Ice milk
- Pudding
- Bananas
- Low fat milk
- Ice cream

This is a clear list and you can see that dairy isn't encouraged at all. If you are someone who drinks a lot of coffee, try cabbage juice or try nettle tea as these are very good at helping you to detox. You may even get to like the taste.

Soft drinks & Juices

- Coke
- Sprite
- Pepsi
- All other colas
- Apple juice
- Orange juice
- Grape juice
- Juices that aren'T Fresh and contain an even a hint of additives

In this day and age, you may have become accustomed to these drinks in your daily life, but you really do need to get out of the habit, even when you have finished the diet since these invariably hide a variety of ingredients, which really are messing with your gut.

Grains

- Cereals
- Muffins
- Breads
- Toast
- Wheat thins
- Sandwiches
- Crackers
- Oatmeal
- Corn
- What
- Cream of wheat

Beans

- Black beans
- Broad beans
- Fava beans
- Carbanzo beans
- Kidney beans
- Horse beans
- Limma beans
- Adzuki beans
- Navy beans
- Red beans
- Pinto beans
- String beans
- White beans
- Snow peas

- Black eyes beas
- Chick peas
- Miso
- Peanuts
- Lentils
- Tofu
- Soybeans

You will find that there are a range of recipes below which you can try but you can also research to make sure that you have a good cross section of recipes to keep you going. Remember, there is no reason why you cannot invent your own recipes, though they must respect the ingredients that are permitted, for the diet to have the full effect.

Paleo Recipes

Banana Omelet

Ingredients:

- 1 banana,
- 3 separated eggs,
- A dash of cayenne pepper,
- Salt & pepper to taste,
- Water,
- Parsley,

Directions:

Cut a banana in half, lengthwise and then cut each of the halves into 3 so that you have 6 pieces at the end. Place these on a baking tray that has been lined with parchment paper and bake until they turn brown or are adequately softened in an oven preheated at 180 degrees. Remember, the riper the banana and the longer it's left in the oven, the drier it will become.

Next, grab a bowl and whisk yolks, pepper, salt and a few spoons of water. Use another bowl to beat the whites until they turn light and fluffy with soft peaks. Fold the yolk mixture you prepared earlier and pour all of it onto a pan placed on medium heat.

Turn over the mixture onto another sheet of paper when the bottoms of the eggs cook, flipping the eggs onto it as you do so. Transfer them into a heated pan and cook for another 3 minutes or until they are browned properly.

After the omelet has cooked, shift it over to a plate and then place the pieces of banana on top of it; sprinkle a little cinnamon and chopped parsley if you want to.

Quick Paleo Pancakes

Ingredients

- 2 eggs,
- ½ cup unsweetened applesauce,
- ½ cup nut butter,
- ¼ teaspoon cinnamon,
- ¼ teaspoon vanilla extract,
- Coconut oil

Mix together all of the ingredients listed (except for the coconut oil) in a bowl, stirring well until a uniform batter is formed. Now, use a spoonful of coconut oil to grease the skillet and spread some of the prepared batter onto it so that a pancake is formed; cook over medium heat before flipping them after 1 minute. Be careful not to wait too long as you may burn them.

Once all of the batter has been used up and pancakes have been cooked, serve them with as many toppings as you have. A few of toppings that may interest you include, chopped apples and cinnamon, real maple syrup, heated blueberries and applesauce.

No-oatmeal

Ingredients

- 1 handful of pecans,
- 1 handful of walnuts,
- ½ to1 teaspoon of ground cinnamon,

- 2 tablespoons flax seed, ground
- A pinch of nutmeg,
- A pinch of ground ginger,
- 1 banana,
- 3 eggs,
- 1 tablespoon almond butter,
- ¼ cup unsweetened almond milk,
- 2 teaspoons pumpkin seeds,
- 1 handful fresh berries

Directions

Add the spices, pecans, walnuts and flax seeds to a food processor and pulse them so a coarse grain is formed. Stop as soon as the grain is turned into powder form and set it aside. Next, whisk almond milk with eggs until it thickens and a loose custard is formed. Blend together the almond butter and mashed banana. Add this banana blend to the custard you prepared earlier and mix.

Add in the nut mixture to his and microwave on the stove until the no-oatmeal reaches a desired level of consistency; the process should only take a few minutes. Finally, sprinkle berries and pumpkin seeds on top and in addition you may add almond milk to this.

Primal Energy bar Recipes

Ingredients

- ½ cup pecans,
- ½ cup slivered almonds,
- ¼ cup unsweetened shredded coconut,
- ¼ cup almond butter; if you want you may use hazelnut, cashew, walnut or pumpkin butter if you want,
- ¼ cup coconut oil,
- ¼ cup almond milk; pulse ¼ cup of almonds in a food processor until a coarse flour is formed,
- 1 ½ teaspoon pure vanilla extract,
- ½ teaspoon raw honey,
- ½ cup protein powder (unsweetened),
- ½ teaspoon sea salt,
- ½ cup blueberries or cranberries,
- ¼ cup unsweetened coconuts

Directions

Use a cookie sheet to toast the nuts and coconut until they turn golden brown in color. Shake the tray at least once while they are being cooked so that they are prepared evenly. Once they're toasted, pour the prepared mixture into a food processor and pulse until the nuts are properly chopped and the entire mixture becomes ground, coarsely.

Use a mixing bowl to melt the almond butter with coconut oil for about 30 seconds before removing from the microwave. Add in the honey, salt and vanilla extract and mix thoroughly. Now take the nut mixture, almond meal and proteins to mix all these thoroughly. Next, add a whole egg & blueberries or cranberries to this, and mix again. Pour this mixture onto an 8x8 pan, which is necessary to keep everything consistent as well as crispier and cook in an oven preheated at 325 degrees for 8 – 10 minutes.

When done, remove from the oven and sprinkle the shredded coconut on top and place it under a broiler until the top develops a golden color. Let the pan cool down for 15 minutes before cutting the energy bar into 12 pieces. If you want you can store it in an airtight container.

Remember that you can cook these in batches so that you always have snacks at the ready should you need them and not want to cheat. This should be a part of your weekly bake or you can choose recipes such as these to make sure that you always have something available when your energy levels are low.

Thai Ground Chicken Salad

Ingredients

- 2 tablespoon lime juice,
- 2 teaspoon minced ginger,
- 1 teaspoon honey,
- 1/8 teaspoon salt,
- 1/8 teaspoon garlic sauce,
- 1 ½ teaspoon virgin olive oil,
- ¼ pound ground chicken,
- 2 cups romaine lettuce shredded,
- ½ cup carrots shredded,
- ¼ cup red onions,
- 2 tablespoons fresh mint leaves,
- 1 tablespoon fresh cilantro,
- 1 – 2 tablespoon chopped cashews.

Directions

Use a small bowl to combine the ginger, honey, limejuice, garlic sauce and salt. Whisk these items by adding olive oil gradually. Take a non-stick pan, place it over medium heat and let it heat until a sprinkle of water sizzles over it. Using an oven mitt, remove the pan from heat and moist it up using an olive oil spray. Place the chicken in the pan and cook it while breaking it up into smaller portions with the help of a spatula; cook the chicken for 5 minutes or until it is no longer pink in color. Remove from the stove and add in a tablespoon of the dressing.

Use a large bowl to combine the carrot, mint, lettuce and cilantro. Toss in the remaining dressing and top it all up with the chicken & nuts. Serve immediately without waiting for it to cool down.

Vegetable Lasagna

Ingredients

- 1 diced onion,
- 700 grams lean meat,
- 3 garlic cloves,
- 4 tablespoon tomato paste,
- 28 oz. diced tomato,
- The following herbs: thyme, sage, mixed Italian herbs, basil and cumin,
- Cinnamon,

- 1 medium eggplant,
- 5 small zucchini,
- 2 tablespoon olive oil,
- ¼ butternut pumpkin

Directions

Preheat an oven to 180 degrees Centigrade.

First, make the mincemeat sauce by frying the garlic & onion in a pan until it turns brown. Stir the minced meat until no more lumps remain. After cooking the meat, return the garlic and onion to pan with the herbs. Add in the tomato paste and cook for another 3 minutes before adding the diced tomatoes and leaving the meat to simmer for 45 minutes.

Use eggplant slices to form a layer at the bottom of an ovenproof dish. On top of these eggplants, use ½ of the mincemeat sauce to form another layer. On top of this layer of meat sauce, spread the pumpkin slices and pour in the remaining sauce on top. Finish off with zucchini slices.

Brush the zucchini slices with olive oil before putting the dish in the oven for 40 minutes or until a spoon goes into the lasagna and comes out dry.

Let the dish cool for 5 minutes.

Chicken Satays with Coriander & Chili

Ingredients

- 6 wooden skewers,
- 1 pound cubed chicken breast,
- ¼ cup lemon juice,
- 1 tablespoon olive oil,
- 1 chopped onion,
- 2 cloves of garlic,
- 1 tablespoon ground turmeric,
- 1 cup coriander leaves,
- 1 tablespoon chili flakes,
- 1 tablespoon garam masala,
- 1 tablespoon coriander seeds,

Directions

Place the onion, lemon juice, garlic cloves, olive oil, coriander, garam masala, and turmeric into a food processor and blend until a very smooth powder is formed. Thread the chicken breasts onto the skewers and place them in a dish; pour the marinade over the chicken until all of it is well soaked. Cover it and place it in the refrigerator for 2 hours.

Preheat the oven to 180 degrees and place the skewers on a tray lined with baking paper. Place the tray in the oven and bake for 30 minutes or until desired level.

Moroccan Chicken Casserole

Ingredient

- 2 – 3 pounds of chicken,
- 1 head cauliflower,
- 1 finely chopped onion,
- 2 tablespoons butter,
- 2 tablespoons ginger root,
- 2 garlic cloves,
- 3 carrots,
- 1 teaspoon paprika,
- 2 teaspoons cumin,
- ½ teaspoon turmeric,
- 1 teaspoon coriander,
- ½ teaspoon cinnamon,
- ¼ teaspoon cayenne pepper,

- 1 red pepper,
- ½ cup diced tomatoes,
- 28 ounce diced tomatoes, undrained,
- 2 teaspoon salt,
- 1 lemon,
- ½ cup cilantro

Directions

Preheat the oven to 375 degrees Fahrenheit. Chop the head of the cauliflower into small pieces and push these pieces into a food processor using a blade. Spread the grated cauliflower onto a 9x13 baking pan. Remember, the base of the casserole is grated cauliflower into rice-like texture.

Sprinkle salt & pepper over the chicken and melt 1 tablespoon of butter in pan over medium to high heat. Add the chicken and let it cook until it browns, which would take 3 – 5 minutes. Next, remove the chicken from the pan and place it somewhere else. Turn the heat down to medium and add ginger, garlic, onion and carrots, cooking until the onions turn soft. Toss in the remaining tablespoon of butter & spices.

Add the can of tomatoes, red pepper, cilantro,

minced parsley and salt, returning the chicken to the pot and letting it simmer for 5 minutes. Pour the mixture over the cauliflower and mix it real nicely until the entire chicken is covered with it. Slice a lemon into some thin slices and lay them on the casserole. Cover the pan with tin foil and place it in the oven for 35 minutes. Remove the foil after 35 minutes and cook for another 25 minutes before serving.

Ivory King Salmon with Chanterelle Mushrooms

Ingredients

- 4 pieces of ivory king salmon steaks,
- ½ pound mushrooms, sliced,
- 4 ounces extra virgin olive oil,
- 16 ounces unsalted organic chicken,
- ½ tablespoon thyme leaves,
- 2 tablespoons minced shallots,
- 1 tablespoon minced garlic,
- 1 tablespoon fresh lemon juice,
- 3 tablespoons whole butter,
- Kosher salt,

- Lemon wedges & parsley sprigs

Directions

Preheat the grill to medium heat; brush the salmon fillets with an ounce of olive oil and season them using kosher salt. Now grill the fish until desired level of doneness is achieved. In the meantime, preheat a sauté pan over high heat and add 3 ounces of oil into it. As soon as the oil becomes very hot, add mushrooms and season them with salt & pepper. Sauté until one of the sides begins to caramelize, which will take approximately 2 minutes. After that, remove the pan from heat and flip the mushrooms so they are cooked on the other side. Empty the mushrooms onto a strainer when done.

Return the pan to heat once again and add a tablespoon of butter to it. Add garlic & shallots, rendering until blonde. Add chicken stock to the pan and let the contents reduce to a sauce. Add the mushrooms back into the pan along with the remainder of butter, gently swirling the pan. Season with salt, pepper & lemon juice and top the fillets with mushroom mixture before serving.

Conclusion

We are well aware of the fact that the moment you saw the signs and symptoms of Hashimoto's appearing in the reactions of your body, you might have gotten really scared. It could seem like a big deal, especially when it starts affecting the outer surface of your body, causing bloating. The moment when you hear people asking you about what happened to your face or why are you avoiding food or why do you avoid sitting with people, you might feel embarrassed going out with your friends who happen to be enjoying life to their fullest. What you need to remember is that people who care for you will understand and it's a good idea to talk to friends and family so that they know what to expect and why you are changing your dietary habits.

You have now taken the first step of unlocking the code of Hashimoto's thyroiditis. You have managed to acquire all the basic information on this disease. You are well aware of what this particular disorder is, what the various causes of the autoimmune disease are, and what you should do in order to get rid of this disease. This book was intended to give you details on the different parts involved in the diagnosis and treatment of

Hashimoto's. These symptoms and indicators will help you to detect the disease just so that you can consult a doctor for the proper medical blood tests. Once you have these, you then know what to expect although it may be a little scary at first. Bear in mind that people manage to live with this disease and that you can manage it better than you may think. You really can.

You have been warned about the various risk factors and misdiagnoses in order for you to analyze yourself better. The treatments mentioned to you have broadened your thought processes as to how you should deal with this disorder. The conventional treatments along with the alternative methods out there have been pointed out for you to help you make a sound decision about your life. The thing is that once you are diagnosed, you find that it makes sense of all the symptoms that you have been suffering from and having a label put on an illness can sometimes help you to make sense of the way that you have been feeling. That's a good thing, because you will know that the depression or dullness that you have been experiencing is normal for people who have been diagnosed with Hashimoto's disease. When that happens, you have a definite way forward.

The next step is to integrate a diet plan, which works with your body in order to fight this disease. If you follow a mainstream nutritional approach, you will just feed Hashimoto's ability to destroy your body even further. In fact, expect to feel bloated, to feel tired and to feel worn out, when in fact you can correct your metabolism and get to a stage where you really do feel good.

Even after reading this book you must, must keep in your mind that you should always consult a professional or your doctor before acting upon any of our suggestions, considering that every human's body is not same nor is everyone's diet plan exactly alike. With the quick recipes given above, you should be seeing that there is a solution to everything, knowing every cloud has a silver lining! So let's not worry ourselves anymore and start working! We sincerely hope that you received all the help you need for cracking the Hashimoto's code.

Thank you again for purchasing this book!

I hope this book was able to help you to manage your thyroid condition and start feeling healthy and vibrant again.

The next step is to apply the information provided in this book on a daily basis. If you can leave feedback for the book, this will help people looking for solutions to their thyroid problems and would be very much appreciated. The information contained in the book is comprehensive and takes into account your lack of information on the disease. It is worthwhile reading it over again because it's a lot of information to take in, but when you understand your illness better, you are then in a position to relate to why so much emphasis has been placed on diet and looking after your digestive system.

I have added several links at the end of the book which readers may find useful and if you are unable to use these as direct links, you will be able to put these into your Internet browser and follow the information contained within those web pages, all of which is backed up in this book and which will help you in your voyage toward improving your health. In particular, you may want to watch the video by the founder of the GAPS diet as this really is helpful and explains the necessity to take diet seriously.

Let's hope that you now have enough

information to try to improve your own Hashimoto's to the extent that you no longer let it control your life, but that you take control – which is how it should be.

References

References: Women 7 times more likely to get Hashimoto's

http://www.healthline.com/health/chronic-thyroiditis-hashimotos-disease#Overview1

Increased chances of Hashimoto's following radiotherapy in neck region.

http://www.ncbi.nlm.nih.gov/pubmed/1514551 1

Article on grounding by Dr. Stephen Sinatra – Heart MD Institute

http://www.heartmdinstitute.com/health-topics/alternative-medicine/grounding-earthing/72-grounding-part

Link required to access the talk by GAPS diet inventor.

https://www.youtube.com/watch?v=hp90Dngf Bwc

Made in the USA
San Bernardino, CA
25 January 2017